To ascertain a better understanding of the following text, it is advised that you read the following books.

The Principles & Philosophy of WEISHENDO

&

**The Burly Man**
Even In Darkness There Is A Light

By

# Zachary E. Lewis

# Salute the Heavens.

致敬的天堂，

The

月亮

Dark

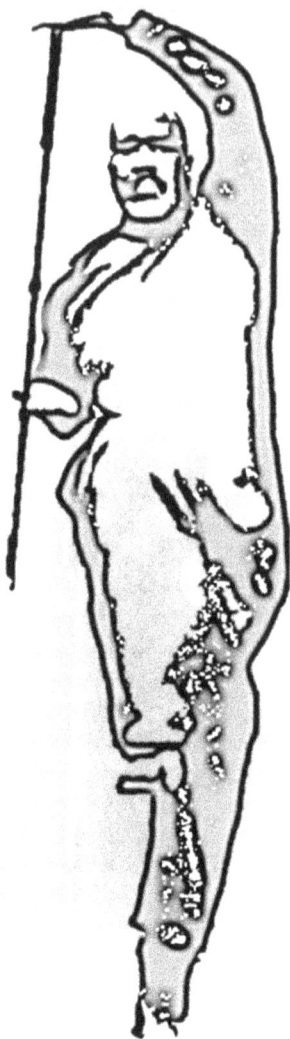

Yin - The Divine Spear

ii

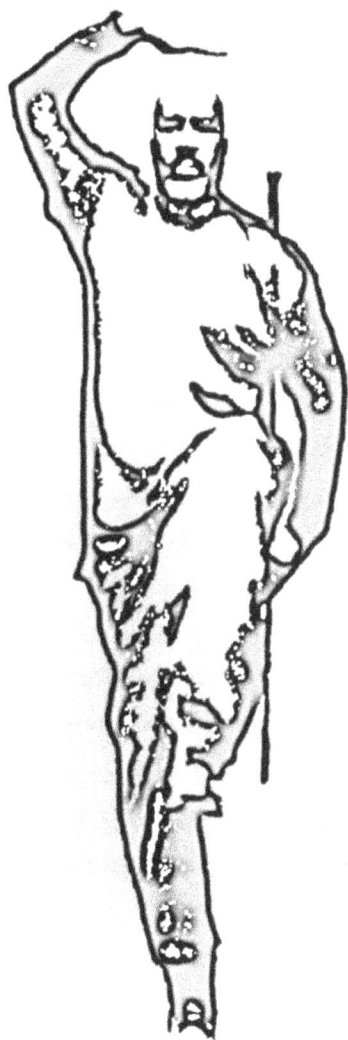

*Embrace the new day.*

迎
接
新
的
一
天

The

太
阳

Light

Yang - The Intrinsic Staff

iii

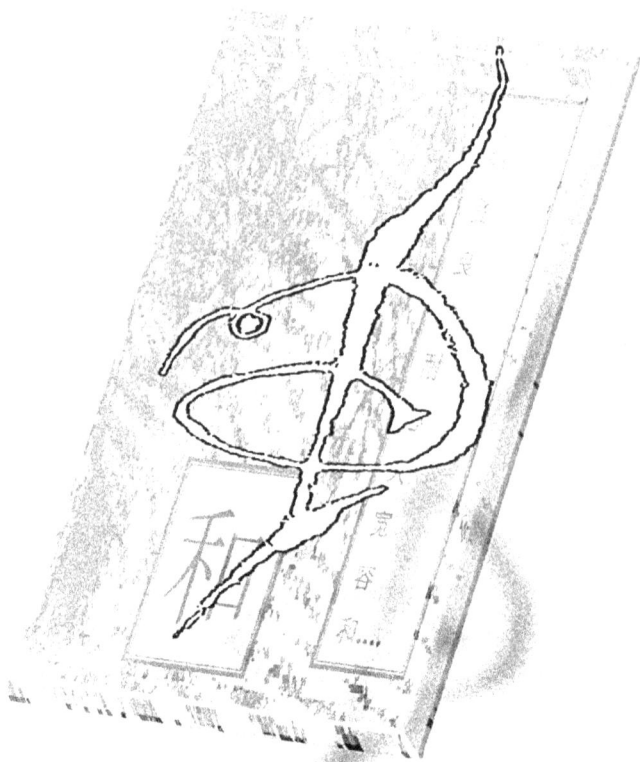

## Disclaimer

Please consult your doctor, or a qualified physical fitness expert, before following this or any fitness plan. The author, nor anyone else involved, will not be held liable for any complications that may occur. The following was developed by Mr. Lewis, and approved by his doctors. By following this régime you do so at your own risk, and accept full responsibility of any problems, difficulties, or injuries.

# The
# Divine Spear
# &
# Intrinsic Staff
# of
# WEISHENDO

Ch'ang     Chieh     Ch'uan

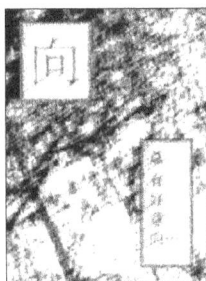

Salute the Heavens Embrace The New Day

By

Zachary E. Lewis

# The
# Divine Spear & Intrinsic Staff

## Of

# WEISHENDO

Ch'ang      Chieh      Ch'uan

### Copyright © 2013 U.S.A.

**Weishendo Publications**
**All Rights Reserved**
**Printed in U.S.A.**

**I.S.B.N. no. 978 - 0 - 578 - 08691 - 0**

**t h e b u r l y m a n @ h o t m a i l . c o m**

*Cover Designs & Interior Illustrations By*

## "The Purest"
# Zachary E. Lewis
*Visit our website @*

# www.weishendopublications.com

# Dedication

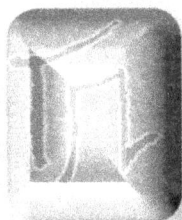 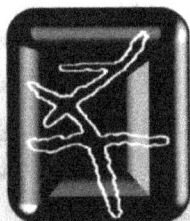 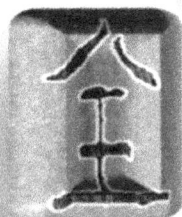

Ch'ang         Chieh         Ch'uan

This book is dedicated to all my Facebook friends and family. The love and support you have shown me throughout my never-ending efforts to raise awareness of autoimmune diseases, will never be forgotten.

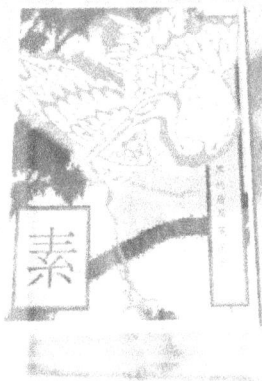

Burly          Man

Salute the Heavens,

and embrace the new day.

# The Preface
## to
# Divine Spear
## &
# Intrinsic Staff

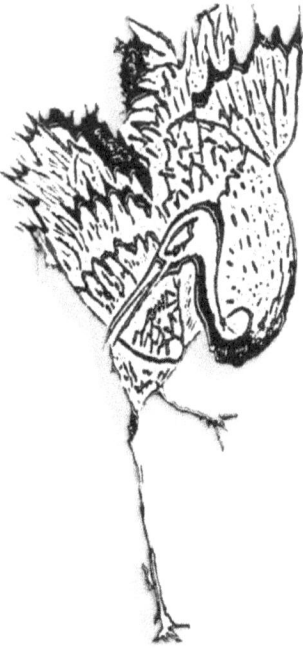

## The Three Precepts
### of
# WEISHENDO

Measurement
Interception
Penetration

In January of 1985, I sat down one Saturday afternoon and watched a martial arts movie. The things that interests me the most was the way in which they moved. Some of them were very simple in application, while others elected to be very elaborate and flashy. This led me to pursue my appetite further. I waited patiently for another movie to come on next week. Once again I noticed the same routine. The elaborate approach to fighting. At this time a spark went off inside me. This is what was to be known as SHEN, or (Spirit of Vitality). This thing called Shen is something we all have, but are not readily aware of. It is the inscrutable operation of **Yin & Yang.**

After watching numerous movies, I went on to purchase my first magazine, which was Inside Kung Fu, September of 1985. In May of 1986, a close friend of mine explained to me what I now know to be Chinese Boxing. In my own ignorance, I called it **"The Open Hand & Closed Fist."** Lacking a Kata or any pre - structuralized technique, it took on a different meaning. The overall task was, to get the job done quickly. With this in mind, I concluded that in order to do what was needed the proponent had to have a clear understanding of, **The 3 Precepts.**

These three significant precepts,
led to this inscrutable conception.

## The

## Principles & Philosophy

## of

# W E I S H E N D O

### Ch'ang

### Chieh

### Ch'uan

After coming across this incredible discovery, I spent the next five years improving my mind, body, and spirit to the utmost of perfection. In doing so, I had achieved a level of peace and harmony with myself and others. This is something we should all strive to achieve.

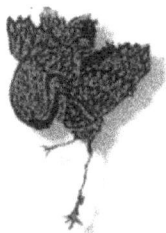

# The Purpose
# of
# W E I S H E N D O
### Ch'ang    Chieh    Ch'uan

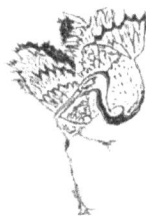

To arrive after a long time, to that which will do equally well, or another way of doing that which some say cannot be done. Thus to advantage both one's self, and others is the way of the ancients. The mind, body, and spirit work in complete harmony. Absolute oneness.

**WEI -** *active and alive. Full of energy, or vigor.*
**SHEN -** *spiritual, and divine, with the unworldly.*
**DO -** *the path or direction in route, and on course.*

# Mu – Shin
## (No - Mint)

*Once set in motion, the mind is completely open and free, taking in everything without effort.  At this point mind, body, and spirit are in complete harmony.  This is known as Mu Shin (**no - mind**).  At the highest level of No-Mind, there is nothing you cannot achieve.*

*   **WEI - SHEN - DO** *is a philosophical way of thinking that is produced by the awareness of mind, body, and spirit. Freedom of movement plus spontaneous and pre-cognitive thought.  From deep within is the cultivation of 3000 years of knowledge, and skill that manifest itself in the flow of what is.  The essence is to flow, while adhering to **Ch'ang Chieh Ch'uan.***

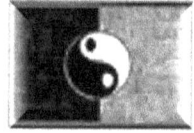

**Yin & Yang**

(一)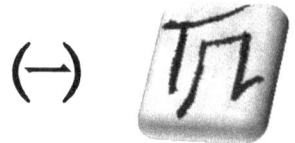

**CH'ANG**

(二)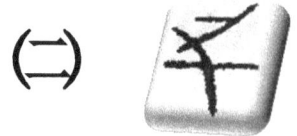

**CHIEH**

(三)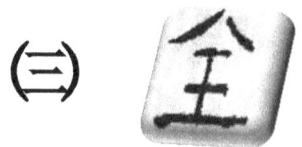

**CH'UAN**

# Ch'ang    Chieh    Ch'uan

*Measurement*    *Interception*    *Penetration*

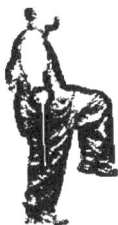 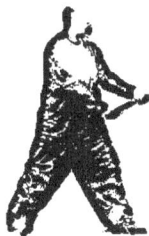 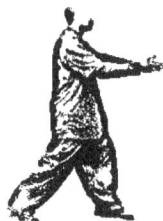

*The principle of **Ch'ang,** is to have the opponent appear to work harder than he has to. Advancing and retreating making his attack or defense to fall on nothing. Thus, giving the illusion that you are too far to defend against, and to close to attack upon. The opponent has been measured.*

*Within intercepting your opponent's offensive, you are now out of the measurement stage. Whatever you do now is the result of mind intent. This is known as **Chieh**. You control the confrontation. You are the stimulus, and the opponent is the response. In this sleight of hand, you control both, the mind (**stimulus**), and the body (**response**). The spirit is the transformation or (**Spirit of Vitality / Shen**).*

*The completion of this auspicious pyramid is **Ch'uan**. This is the mind, body, and spirit making actual contact with the opponent. In **The Realm of Combat**, you have **(One):** Approached and solved the problem of distance between you and your opponent. **(Two):** Intercepted your opponent's futile attack. **(Three):** Successfully launched your attack, and released your own Shen upon the assailant without effort.*

# The Ode To Spear & Staff

*To* be de-void of **detention**,

does not imply **retention**,
it opens up the opportunity,
to **intention**.

*To* be de-void of **aggression**,

does not imply **repression**,
it opens up the opportunity,
to **suppression**.

*To* be de-void of **oppression**,

does not imply **regression**,
it opens up the opportunity,
to **ascension**.

# Declarations
# of
# Intent

Declaración de intenciones

## #One
### i

*T*he will to *fulfill,*

*or advance in any task is lost,*

*if you lack the effort to do so.*

## #Two
### ii

*T*he slightest *actions,*

*can reveal the most yielding,*

*of precepts.*

# Rising Above

你一定感到好像　豪放状态是心理的本质　你是像风自然光线　生活之前你自己　你必须愿意躺在你的　清空你自己。忘掉输赢

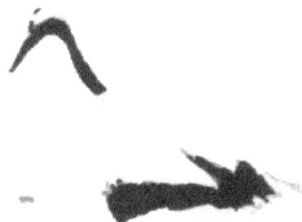

Empty yourself. Forget about winning or losing.

You must be willing to lay your life, before yourself.

You must feel as though you are light like the wind.

An uninhibited state of mind is of the essence.

# Stepping Stones

在正确的方向一步

可以改变一切的在世界

即使是一个小巨人的世界中

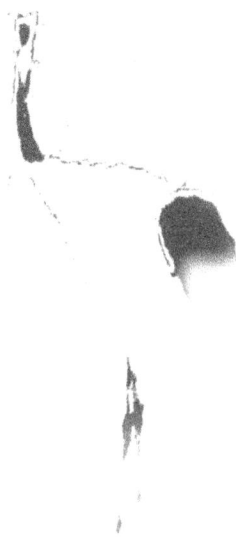

One step in the right direction,

can make all the difference, in the world.

Even if it is a small one, in a world of giants.

# Acknowledgement
*Principles of Applied Philosophies*

After writing **The Principles and Philosophy of WEISHENDO**, it was clear to me this doctrine would one day be a benefit to others. What I didn't realize was how vital, and beneficial it was to my daily life. I was able to incorporate my principles into almost any situation by substituting a word, a phrase, or concept where applicable. This gave me the advantage I was missing for so many years, assimilation.

To achieve this I had to adapt, change, assimilate, and transcend unconsciously at will, without using any force. The combative strategies I developed from practicing martial arts were useful in fighting both illnesses, along with the assimilation of my **Principles of Applied Philosophies**. It was an enigmatical complex of math cognitive equations, that took over 20 years to comprehend, and develop.

Now that I'm ready to put my theories to the test. Can these equations work against something as multifaceted, and incurable as an autoimmune disease? Given the challenge, this book was written for just this purpose. The assimilation of principles, and philosophies, which will give you optimal performance of the latter; through the guidance of **Measurement, Interception, and Penetration.**

# THE PUREST
## Zachary E. Lewis
### a.k.a. The Burly Man

Mr. Lewis story starts out on January of 1985, as he sat down one Saturday afternoon to watch a martial arts movie. Six years later, he wrote down detailed notes of what would be the foundation of his principles and philosophy, which he called **W E I S H E N D O** (*way of the active spirit*). Having done what few people could only dream of doing, he went a step further. Mr. Lewis spent the next seventeen years trying to understand the answers to a question that was given to him from his late grandmother Mamie Turner. On December 21$^{st}$, 2007, everything started to make sense. Putting mind, body, and spirit into a meditative state for eight months, on July 31$^{st}$, 2008 Mr. Lewis had reached the end of his journey by publishing, **"The Principles & Philosophy of WEISHENDO."** But for Burly Man, the journey had only just begun.

On June 17$^{th}$ 2009, Mr. Lewis had his first of many ER visits to the hospital. Eight months later on February 12$^{th}$, 2010, he was diagnosed with Polymyositis. On August 25$^{th}$, of 2010, he was diagnosed with Lupus. Both are incurable Auto-Immune Diseases. During this time, Mr. Lewis wrote a daily journal, which he called, **"The Burly Man"** (*which tells the events that led to his diagnosis of Polymyositis*). Having already written **"The Principles & Philosophy of WEISHENDO"** (*to help him better understand himself and others,*) he took something negative and turned it into something positive. Mr. Lewis used his techniques to help him fight against the illnesses that plague his mind, body, and spirit. With the edition of his third book **"The Divine Spear & Intrinsic Staff"** (*which is a special exercise book that he has developed to help him maintain a better quality of life,*) he has taken his art form to a completely new level by adapting it for others. As quoted from this very book. "The will to fulfill, or advance in any task is lost, if you lack the effort to do so."

# Contents

# Appendix pg. 287

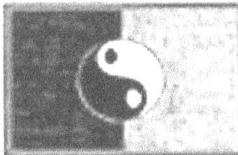

它不是理论的赢得每场战斗，作为先决条件赢得了战争

It is not a theory of winning every battle, as a prerequisite, to winning the war....

# Chapter

# 1.

## Motion
## &
## Energy

### The Crane Form
### Simplified Daily Exercise Routine

---

*A trapped mind is a spirit that is confined inside an abode,*
*that is often led to believe, or fooled by illusions of grandeur.*

*Free the mind, and the vessel becomes replenished,*
*thus allowing the spirit to ascend...*

*A free mind is an absolute mechanism....*
*Refined... tuned... and rhythmically, resolved....*

---

The Purest
*A.D.* 2008

# Releasing Energy

While in the flow, an individual must associate with numerous arrays of techniques; or methods that adhere to **economy of motion, and simplicity**. Therefore, it is essential when releasing energy, (**or Jing**) the entire body must be involved in one continuous motion. Such power originates at the **balls of the rear foot.** It must travel through the body for it to be used efficiently. The path of true enlightenment goes as such.

1. Fingers
2. Shoulders     **Upper Body**
3. Spine
4. Waist
5. Legs          **Lower Body**
6. Foot

*Advanced Lead*

*Rear Ft.*

R.     L.

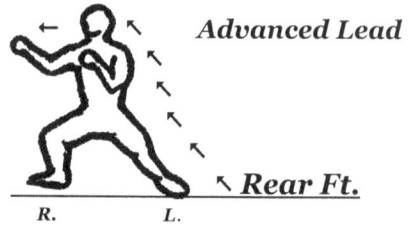

There is also the angle of trajectory. The quickest path between two points is a straight line. In theory, the further a strike has to travel the more power and speed it can generate. In the case of the offensive application, the advanced lead is positioned in front of the body, and travels down the center line. Because of the position the lead takes, it will land quicker, and accurately. As the lead hand moves forward, the push off from the rear leg will generate the necessary speed and power. This will add to the acceleration of the strike.

$$F = ma$$

**1.** The advance of the lead arm.

**2.** The lead leg rises slightly.

**3.** The push off from the rear ft.

*Gravity* ↓

*Rear ft.*

*Floor* ↑

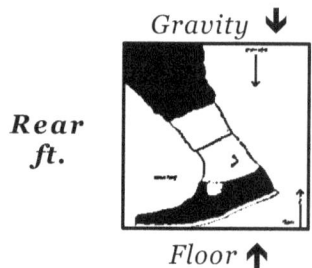

With the left foot forward and the right hand thrusting, the body will work against itself. But, with the right foot forward and the right hand thrusting, equal force is applied. This would most definitely suggest that the dominant side or stronger side of the body should lead in all releasing acts. (***There are exceptions to this***).

# Transferring Energy

The maximum transfer of energy requires the most efficient use of force producing motions in the body, and the maximum range of motion at the point of contact. If a fighter doesn't go through an extreme range of bodily motion before he releases his energy, the result will be a poor exertion of body motion.

1. The best transfer of energy occurs from large muscle groups, in the direction of smaller muscle groups.

    a. The advanced lead is a combination of large, and small muscles acting in the same direction.

2. Any transfer of energy from one form to another, is easily done with economy of motion, and simplicity of efficiency. The smooth transfer of energy is released.

    b. The proper sequence of motion is known as the **Kinetic Chain.**

3. Any motion that involves excess tension or excess muscular contraction will use inefficient energy. This will result in the decrease of total energy.


**Potential Energy** - *Any amount of energy that is stored, and made readily available to the work of which is about to be done.* <u>**(The pre-stage of any strike or kick is non - telegraphic).**</u>


**Kinetic Energy** - *Any amount of energy that is in motion and non – prohibited has momentum, of which energy is applied during the work.* <u>**(The post - stage is continual cognitive work).**</u>

## Note....

*The amount of energy in a specific object will never die, but there are times when it can be focused or redirected.*

# Issuing Energy

**The Advanced Lead** is executed without any forewarning. Thrusting the hand before the body, everything follows in one smooth motion. The concept behind this is **simplicity.** You advance your lead hand from the true guard position, with your lead hand in the position of that which protects any part of the whole during attack. In the on-set, there is no windup, you advance from the true guard position and penetrate through the target.

*The advanced lead can be very useful as long as, you remember some of the basic principles of motion.*

1. When you use the lead, remain calm and relaxed. The upper back and shoulders should be used for close range strikes. There should be little or no movement at all from the shoulder. **(Concentrate on issuing energy).**

2. Penetrate past the point of impact. Do not focus or tense your arm. When punching, use the triceps muscles, not the biceps.

3. In the on-set, there is no windup. The forearm serves as the defensive guard for the strike. The elbow serves a dual role. The elbow initiates the driving force, and can deflect or change directions.

4. As you move forward, your rear hand comes back to protect your face, a.k.a. **(the guard hand).** The final surge comes from the wrist of the lead hand. In the pre-stage, the wrist is relaxed, but at the final execution, it turns up and the last 4 knuckles of the hands are used to strike.

# Kinetic Energy

You must always adhere to three key factors during the execution of the advanced lead.  **One**: Always occupy the centerline of your opponent, as you will penetrate his defense, and intercept his offense. **Two**: Facing your opponent must incorporate a stance that will appear non- threatening to him. **Three**: The economy of your motion in the use of the advanced lead must be simple and direct.

***To properly execute the advanced lead,
you must thoroughly understand Kinetic Energy.***

1. The length or the distance your hand must travel should not be over extended. Upon contact, your lead elbow should still be at an acute angle. ***Not more than 90 degrees.*** **(Sharp)**

2. The perpendicular or parallel distance from the fulcrum, is a vertical or horizontal fist. Your elbow is the originator of thus said force. **Equivalence is the simplicity**, **of productive magnitude.**

3. Your energy must be able to flow freely without any alteration to its rotation.  If your elbow were to be motor set, it would rob the flow of its continuity. Stationary but not stagnant is the key.

*The kinetic energy of a body is the energy due to its motion. The faster a body moves the more kinetic energy it possesses. When a body stops moving, the energy is lost. This is readily seen in the advanced lead.*

# *Law of Inertia*
## (#1) - I

**N**ewton's first law of motion goes as such. A body continues to move forward or remain at rest unless an unbalanced force acts upon it. In short, it will continue to move a considerable distance until a force is applied to alter its motion. If there is no initial force, it will not move.

## *Example: #1*

### *This holds true to the advanced lead in attack.*

**I~a** *The originator of the force to move the hand is the elbow.*

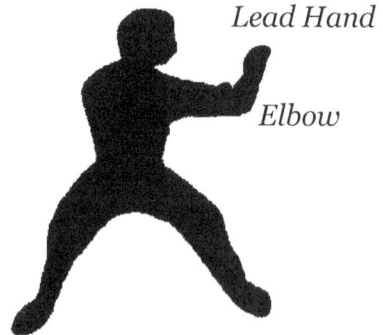

*Lead Hand*

*Elbow*

**II~a** *The hand will move forward, with a slight flexing of the appropriate muscles.*

**III~a** *As the initial motion is made, the elbow will drive the hand.*

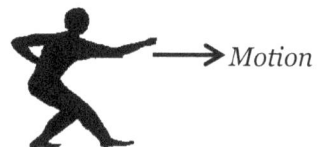

→ *Motion*

With an increase in speed, the greater the mass in any object, the greater its inertia will be as well. The measure of inertia in a body is mass. In the application of the advanced lead, the elbow has the most mass at this point in **space, time, and reality.**

# Law of Acceleration
## (#2) - II

**N**ewton's second law of motion goes as such. The acceleration of an object is directly proportional to the force causing it, in the same direction as the force, and is inversely proportional to the mass of the object. The product of a force, and the time over which it acts is known as impulse. (**F=ma**)

## Example: #2

*A fighter thrusting his body forward to achieve acceleration.*

**I~b** *An increase in momentum occurs when the force causing the increase, is applied in the same direction of the momentum.*

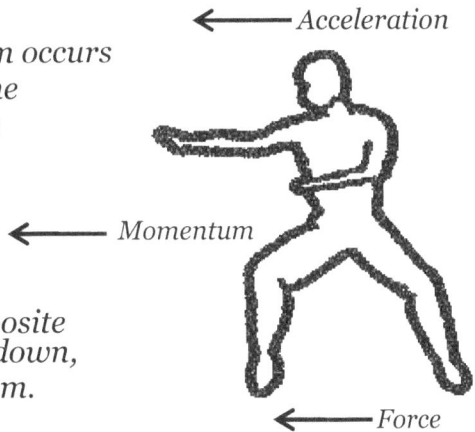

←——— *Acceleration*

←——— *Momentum*

**II~b** *Force applied in the opposite direction can also slow down, or decrease in momentum.*

←——— *Force*

**III~b** *Thus the dominant or strong side should lead to create equal force. Execute with the method that yields the greatest momentum.*

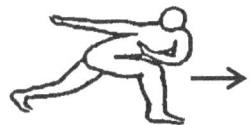

*Opposite Direction*

——→

**Note.... This does not hold true, to every medium of motion. Address accordingly.**

# Law of Reaction
## (#3) - III

**N**ewton's third law of motion goes as such. For every action, there is an equal and opposite reaction. When a body exerts force on another, the second will in turn exert an equal and opposite force on the initial.

## Example: #3

*This is seen when the rear foot pushes against the ground.*

**I~c** *Likewise, the ground pushes against the foot. Without the forward push of the ground against the rear foot, the kinetic energy and forward thrust would not be possible.*

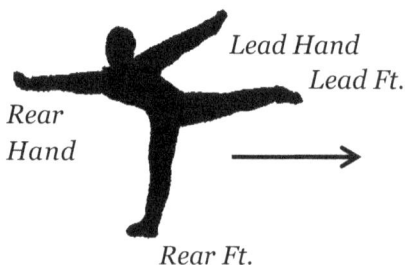

Lead Hand
Lead Ft.
Rear Hand
Rear Ft.

# Moment of Inertia
## (#4) - IV

Once set in motion, spinning bodies tend to keep their relative spinning motion. As with linear motion, force applied to start or stop a spinning object is related to its mass.

**I~d** *A ball rotating on the end of a long string is harder to stop than a ball on a much shorter string.*

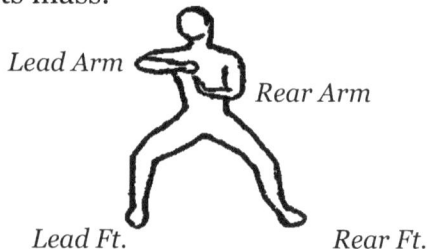

Lead Arm
Rear Arm
Lead Ft.
Rear Ft.

# Change of Inertia
## (#5) - V

In the human body, the mass distribution
can be altered by changing the body position.

### This is known as the change of inertia.

**I-e** *A fighter is capable of moving the lead leg and hand more rapidly, when it is in a flexed position, as opposed to being fully extended.*

**II-e** *When the appendage is closer to the axis and flexed, the moment of inertia is less. The rule for linear motion also applies for rotary motion.*

# Angular Momentum
## (#6) - VI

The measure of the force needed to initiate or halt motion is known as momentum. Any object in angular motion has momentum. The same is true for an object in linear motion.

**I-f** *Linear momentum is the product of mass and velocity.*

**II-f** *Angular momentum is the product of the angular equivalents of mass and velocity.*

**(Moment of Inertia & Angular Velocity)**

# Action and Reaction
## (#7) - VII

Yang
*right*
*hand*

Yin
*left*
*hand*

**Basic Stance pg. 82**

yang          yin

Right Leg

Left Leg

Lead Ft.

Rear Ft.

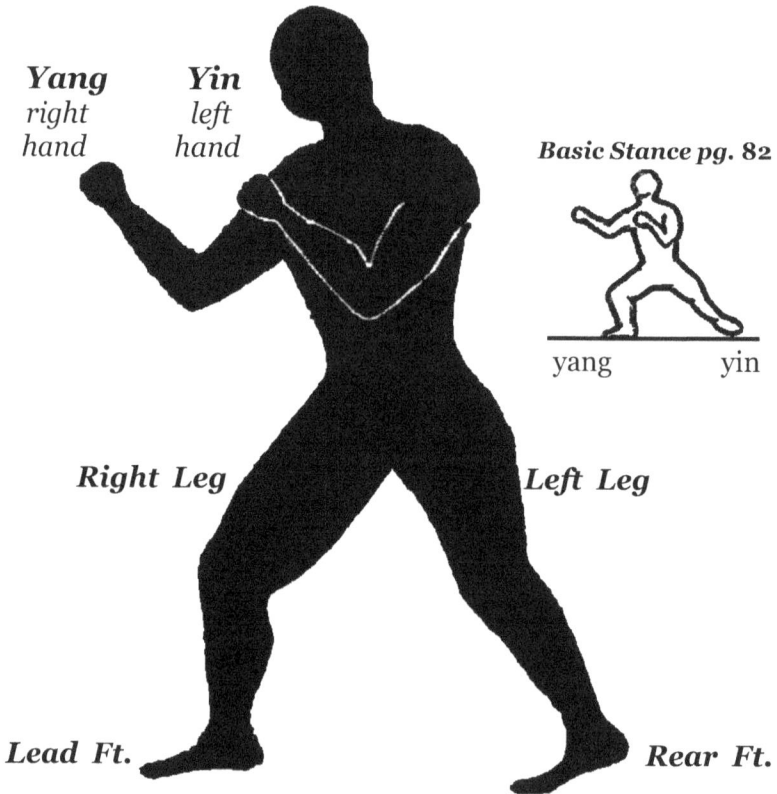

**I-g**  *The force of angular motion is torque. The torque acting on the legs, is an equal and opposite torque acting on the rest of the body.* **(I.e. the rear & lead uppercut in angular velocity).**

**II-g**  *The trunk segment is less because the latter* **(the push off of the rear leg)** *is much greater. The change in angular velocity of the arms, and trunk in forward upward motion is slightly visible.*

# Angular Velocity
## (#8) - VIII

When the arms swing horizontally across in front of the body, the trunk produces an opposing action on the rest of the body in the transverse plane.

**I~h** *There are times when action and reaction of specific body parts are unwanted or unneeded.*

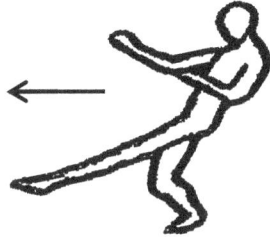

The rotation of the pelvis and legs about a vertical axis produces an undesired reaction of the upper trunk in the opposite direction, if not controlled in some other method.

**I~h** *The arms should move in opposition to the leg movement.*

**II~h** *This absorbing motion produces the counter twist.*

**III~h** *This will cancel the response of the body on the legs.*

**IV~h** *The action is doubled as the legs rotate about the axis.*

| #1 Kai - *neutralize* | #2 Ho - *seize* | #3 Fa - *advance* |
|:---:|:---:|:---:|
| 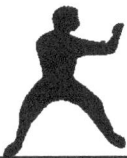 | 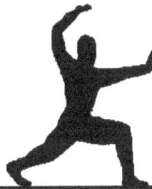 | 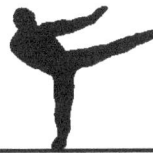 |

# Centripetal Force
## (#9.) - IX

*When one swings a weight around on the end of a wire, the force causing the weight to change direction constantly, is known as centripetal force.*

**I-i**  *There is a force, which moves the object at right angles.*

**II-i**  *Because of the latter, it will rotate in a circular path.*

**III-i**  *The amount of centripetal force used to keep an object rotating in a circular path is directly proportional to its mass.*

**IV-i**  *If you double the mass, the centripetal force is doubled.*

**V-i**  *Shorten the radius and maintain present speed of the latter.*

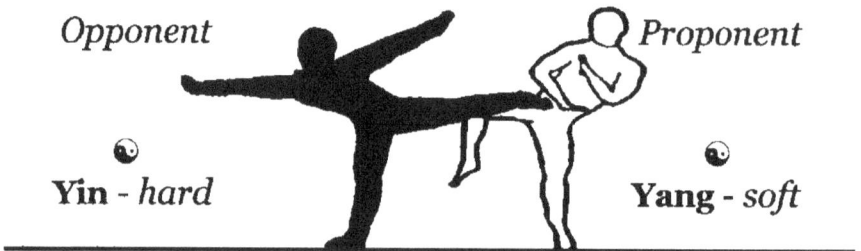

Opponent

Proponent

**Yin** - *hard*

**Yang** - *soft*

## Note....

**The latter will cause centripetal force to increase. This force is displayed, in any spinning kick or strike when rotation is applied.**

# Centre of Gravity

**I~j** When all the forces acting on a body equal zero, equilibrium is achieved.

**Ia~j** The centre of gravity will remain unchanged as long as the body does not change shape. If you change shape or the position of the body, the centre will be offset. Such knowledge is needed when finding the perfect base.

**IIb~j** The effort to control balance in an unfavorable position is known as one of the basic motor skills. Standing on one foot while executing a kick, or in the application of the lunge will demonstrate this.

**IIIc~j** When the application of the latter is displayed, the effort is called static balance. The only time that your body does not adjust is when it is in a state of complete repose. The intent is to execute with minimum motion.

**IVd~j** If you lower the centre of gravity, this will increase the stability of the body. Because of the angular displacement of gravity & centre, the increased stability is greater. The wider the base, the greater the support will be.

**Ve~j** If the stance is wider than the breath of the pelvis, the legs will take on a slanting position. Too wide of a stance is not advised. The wider the stance the less control you have in shuffling your feet. (**I.E. momentum**)...

# Chapter #1 Review

Releasing Energy

Transferring Energy

Issuing Energy

Kinetic Energy

---

Law of *Inertia*

Law of *Acceleration*

Law of *Reaction*

Change of *Inertia*

Moment of *Inertia*

Angular *Momentum*

Action and *Reaction*

Angular *Velocity*

Centripetal *Force*

Centre of *Gravity*

# Efflorescence

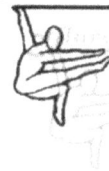

The beauty of Shen is to arrive at that which some say cannot be done, or to accomplish that which appears to be of an acquired task, which seems effortless in execution.

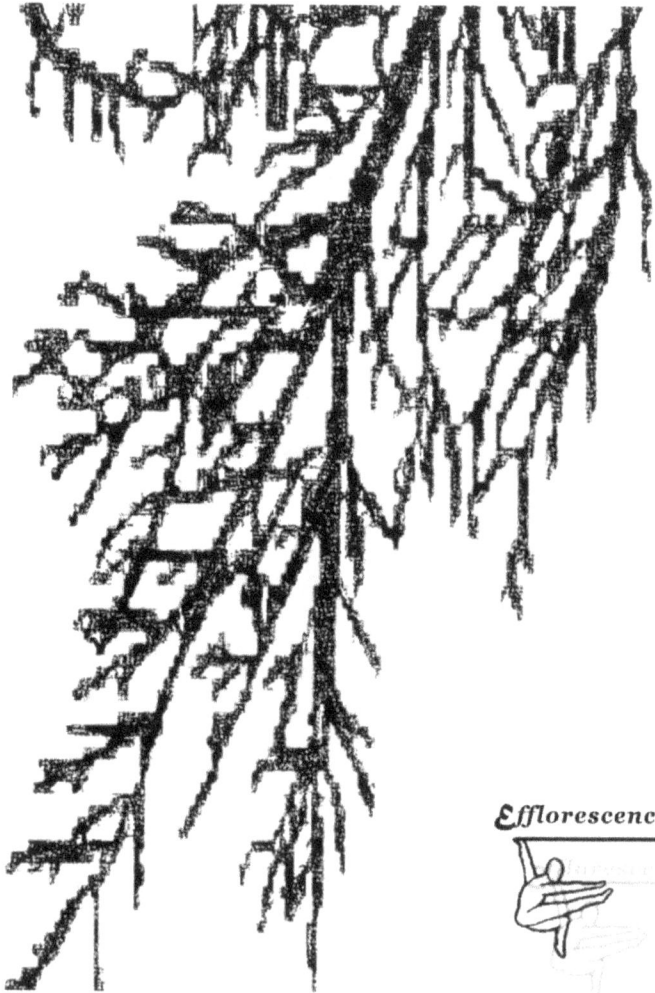

Efflorescence

# Chapter 2.

## The Divine Spear
## &
## The Intrinsic Staff

### The Crane Form Part One
### Simplified Daily Exercise Routine

---

**The Salute:** *A gracious bird salutes the heavens.*

**The Embrace:** *A Poignant bird embraces the new day.*

---

*When we push the limits to exceed them,*
*we do so not,*
*to exhaust them totally, without residual.....*

# The Crane Form

The greatest advantage to **The Divine Spear & Intrinsic Staff** (or *DSIS*) is that no equipment of any kind is needed, other than a staff or simple walking stick. The exercise can be performed with or without a staff at any time, or any place. Clothing should be light and loose fitting to help aid your performance. Although a good connection to the ground will enable a better flow of balance, and energy, shoes are optional. The only thing I would recommend is to either perform the movements in the morning, or at night before you go to bed. The exercise is best suited to help you function throughout your day, or as a relaxing agent to transition you into a night time regiment. Alternate between morning, midday, or early evening.

The Divine Spear & Intrinsic Staff can be thought of, as a corporal aspect of **WEI-SHEN-DO**, with the goal of better physical control and relaxation. Looking deeper into the purpose of **DSIS, (*Divine Spear & Intrinsic Staff*)** it's not just a series of exercises, but a unique blend of postures and poses. It is at its best, the beginning stages toward a better quality of life, and wellness. With the variance of each segment, you are not bound to perform each one as written. This text serves only as a guideline. Our purpose is to promote fundamental movement, whether it's bed ridden or wheelchair bound. There is always a beneficial gain, as you advance your daily activity.

*The main emphasis is on overall well-being, through a relaxed transitory, and tensionless state of mind. As you explore the benefits of The Divine Spear & Intrinsic Staff if only for a general feeling of wellness, you will find with regular practice it will greatly improve muscular tone. Also, help to increase suppleness, and improve the circulatory system of the body.*

*There are two key points of interest,*
*one must remember when practicing.*

**1.** **Execute every movement slowly, and gracefully. Avoid stress in motion.** *A good deal of practice is needed before some of the more advanced poses can be achieved. You are looking for sangfroid,* (**poise**), *and suppleness* (**agility**), *along with consequent relaxation of mind, body, and spirit. Do not exhaust yourself or attempt advanced poses before you are ready.*

**2.** **Correct breathing is vital to each exercise segment. (Residual Constants of Natural Breathing).** *Go through each pose, and try to hold the position until it starts to feel uncomfortable. Remembering to breathe, each one is designed to enhance a particular part of the body. Breathing is relaxed and not forced, as each transition into a movement is achieved without pressure.*

## *A*uthors *N*ote

*The four exercise segments can be done individually or altogether. Within each segment, the movements can be broken down through their breathing order, or isolated through their motions. As you breathe in it is considered insubstantial, or as you breathe out it is considered substantial, or vice versus. Unlike conventional methods, you will be performing the segments during times of great physical stress, in an effort to increase your daily and future activity. Whereas, normal exercise methods would suggest you refrain from any activity until you are physically able to do so.*

# Principles

When using the spear or staff, if should be thought of,
as if it were an extension of the mind, body, and spirit.

When executing the intricate movement patterns,
you must go through linear & circular movements.

The entire body should be used, as a single mechanism,
controlling the spear or staff.

The true purpose of the spear or staff,
is to enhance the internal as well as the external.

The front hand must be considered yang,
while the rear hand is yin, or vice versa.

Energy must pass through the entire shaft to the tip,
which comes from the bottoms of the feet.

All movement should be soft, relaxed,
and held with a calm and quiet nature.

Each form should be held, until a maximum state of
equilibrium is maintained, to promote your balance.

# Precepts

For the purest, it is a matter of being spontaneous.
To win, you must be direct and unattainable....


The force applied is like water rushing down a mountain.
The limits of such actions can be unlimited.


It is not a theory of winning every battle,
as a prerequisite, to winning the war....


Being victorious is about being varied. The methods
are so unlimited that they travel to infinity....


To be without any plausible means of ever coming to an end,
you have reached a state of which is almost indefinable.


Having influence is like breaking a glass.
The structure and the shape must change....


The Purest, is established by his diversion,
which is his ability to be centered, by applying division.


The application of any motion is performed to the
maximum, by the means of not being seen, felt or even heard....

# Natural Breathing

**Breathe In: B. I.**  
Yin

**Breathe Out: B. O.**  
Yang

---

**THE SALUTE :** *A gracious bird salutes the heavens.* **B.I.**

**THE EMBRACE :** *A poignant bird embraces the new day.* **B.O.**

---

*Breathe-in* _expand_ **(yin)**          *Breathe-out* _contract_ **(yang)**

| Exercise Segment | Face East | Face South | + Centre | Face West | Face North |
|---|---|---|---|---|---|
| **I.** | | 1. B. I.<br>2. B. O.<br>3. B. I.<br>4. B. O.<br>5. B. I.<br>6. B. O. | | | |
| **II.** | 7. B. I.<br>8. B. O.<br>9. B. I.<br>10. B. O.<br>11. B. I. | | | | |
| **III.** | | | | 12. B. O.<br>13. B. I.<br>14. B. O.<br>15. B. I.<br>16. B. O. | |
| **IV.** | 17. B. I.<br>18. B. O.<br>19. B. I.<br>20. B. O. | | | | |

There are two basic breathing patterns. The first one is called **"Normal Breathing or Natural Breathing,"** (*Breathing* - chi / *energy or life*) because it is the way we breathe normally. The stomach expands as we breathe in, and contracts as we breathe out. *When you breathe in it is **yin**. When you breathe out it is **yang**.* During Normal Breathing, the stomach expands on all four sides. As you Inhale, gather the chi (<u>breath</u>) into the **tan tien**. As you exhale the stomach contracts from all four sides again. The chest, diaphragm, and pelvic contract, lifting upward as they push air out.

When you are excited, exhausted, or exercising, you will find yourself breathing in reverse**. "Reverse Breathing"** is more difficult to practice than Normal Breathing. For this reason, we will focus on normal breathing. When Abdominal Breathing is done correctly, the expanding and contracting movements from the stomach massage your internal organs, thus improving their circulation.

Stand in **"The Ready Position,"** and make yourself relaxed as possible. (*Place the left hand in a **proximal position** in front of the chest. Holding the staff or spear in your right hand, place it behind the back of the right shoulder with the tip pointing up*). Taking in a couple of deep breaths, this is done to calm your mind. Breathe in slowly through the nose, and touch the roof of your mouth with your tongue, remembering not to bite down or grind the teeth. As you exhale do the same. Repeat the sequence as desired. Do not use your stomach muscles, to force your breath. Remain calm and reserved. (*The best time to do this is when you first wake up, or before you go to bed*).

When out of breath, people tend to breathe through their mouth, because the mouth's opening is larger than the nose. Breathing in such a manner is not wrong, but the throat will dry quickly. The breath becomes light, and shallow, which causes the **Microcosmic Channel** to cut off. In your daily practice concentrate on breathing through the nose. Place the tongue on the roof of the mouth, and try not to bite down with your teeth. To do so would be a negative gesture, which leads to tension and strain.

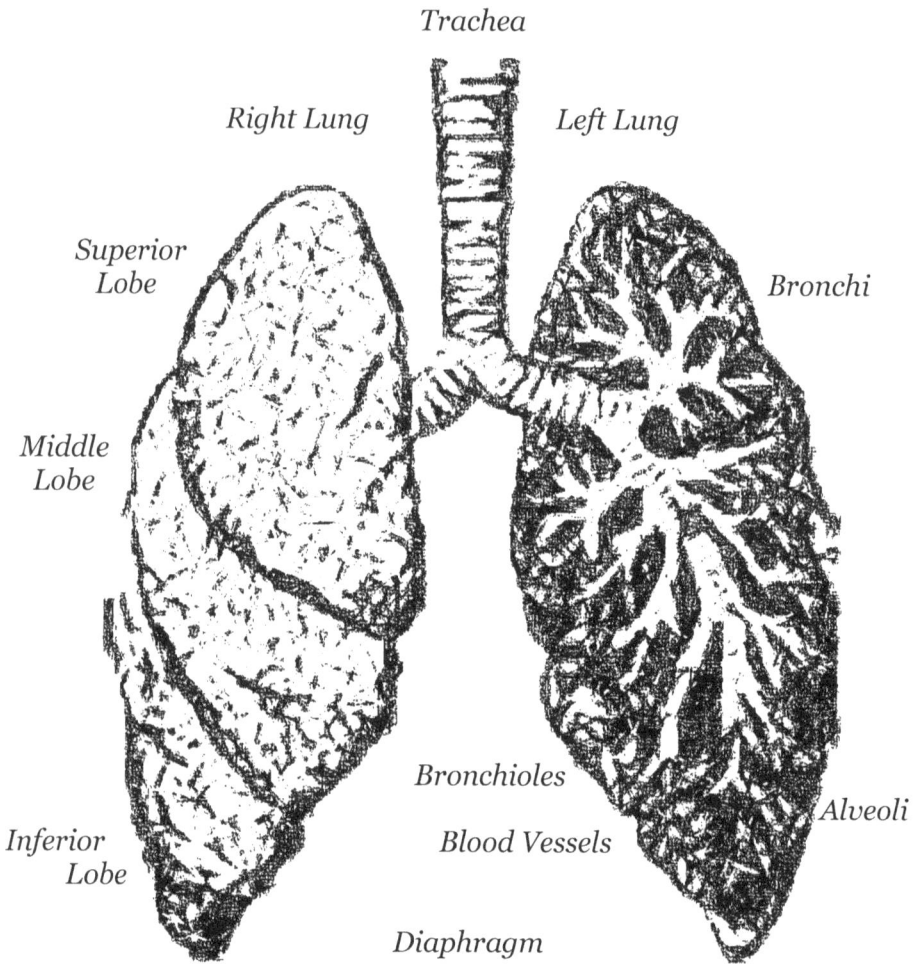

Trachea

Right Lung

Left Lung

Superior Lobe

Bronchi

Middle Lobe

Bronchioles

Alveoli

Inferior Lobe

Blood Vessels

Diaphragm

Although **Myositis** and other Autoimmune Diseases like **Lupus** cause muscle weakness and fatigue, physical activity is crucial to overcoming these conditions. Lack of movement can bring on stiffness, and low energy. You don't have to engage in high-impact workouts or strenuous activities. Simple exercises such as **Walking, Stretching, The Crane Form, Tai Chi, Qi Gong, and Yoga** are enough to improve your flexibility and fight tiredness. Make a conscious effort to incorporate some form of physical activity into your daily routine, as it will stimulate your lungs. A good exercise program consists of 30 minutes of physical activity, at least three to four times a week.

*Crane comes from the Angelo-Saxon, Cran.*
*" To Cry Out "*

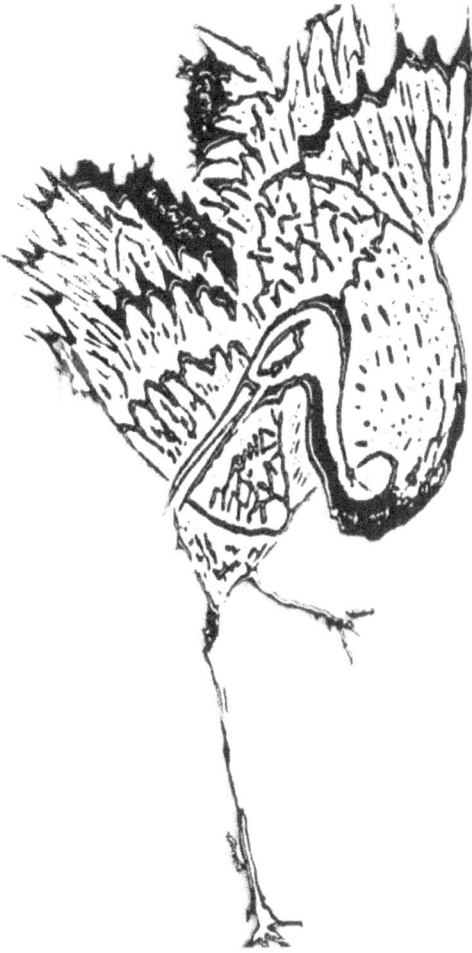

# Meditation

When meditating, you should focus on a place that is calm and serene. Set aside time to meditate so you will not be bothered by others. It has been said often that, *"The amateur meditates to relax, whereas the professional relaxes to meditate."* Thus, we relax to meditate. The environment and meditative posture will help you to reach complete relaxation. Being that there are 3 primary postures for meditation, we will focus on the one that is the most effective. **Standing Meditation.**

**"Standing Meditation"** is the ability to move without moving. It may appear as if you are not doing anything, but the physical and mental effects are equal to almost any physical exercise. In this motionless posture, one should observe changes in energy from inside, and outside the body. Besides building leg strength, standing opens the channels of the hands and feet. In the standing posture, chi comes in from the crown of the head, and the soles of the feet.

*Meditate in the ready position, as this will help you to focus your chi.*

# THE CRANE FORM

<u>**THE SALUTE:**</u> *A gracious bird salutes the heavens.*

<u>**THE EMBRACE:**</u> *A poignant bird embraces the new day.*

---

### Appellations
### Exercise Segment 1.

#### face South

1. Insightful Crane sweeps to the south.
2. Secure the right wing.
3. Crane spreads his right wing open.
4. Secure the left wing.
5. Crane spreads his left wing open.
6. Powerful bird holds up the sky.

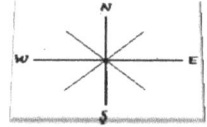

---

### Exercise Segment 2.

#### face East

7. Advance to release.
8. Immaculate bird strikes its prey.
9. Diligent Crane rotates its beak.
10. Divine bird looks 2 the heavens.
11. Ambitious Crane looks for food.

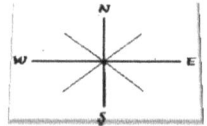

---

### Exercise Segment 3.

#### face West

12. Heroic bird stretches his wings.
13. Uncanny Crane stomps his foot.
14. Fearless bird grabs a fish.
15. Poignant bird embraces the new day.
16. Insightful Crane sweeps to the west.

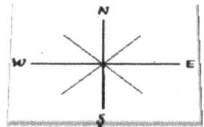

---

### Exercise Segment 4.

#### face East

17. Lofty bird goes down under.
18. Crane spreads his right wing open.
19. Angry Crane flaps his wings.
20. The agile bird points to the south.

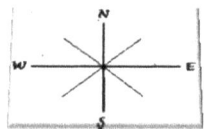

---

As the exercise completes,
you return to the originator.

**THE SALUTE:** *A gracious bird salutes the heavens.*
**THE EMBRACE:** *A poignant bird embraces the new day.*

---

# PERPETUAL MOTION

When your weight is placed more heavily on your right side,

the right side of your body will be substantial (**positive or yang**).

Whereas the left side will be insubstantial (**negative or yin**).

~~~~~~~~~~~~

When your weight is placed more heavily on your left side,

the left side of your body will be substantial (**positive or yang**).

Whereas the right side will be insubstantial (**negative or yin**).

~~~~~~~~~~~~

### The Mathematical Equation

#1 Occupy your **space - (S)**

#2 Utilize your **time - (t²)** $$\frac{S\,t^2}{\infty} = R$$

#3 While being **realistic - (R)**

# "Opening Movement"

*The Salute:* A gracious bird salutes the heavens.

*The Embrace:* A poignant bird embraces the new day.

---

| ⬤=0% | ◐=TOES | ◑=HEEL | ◯=100% |
|:---:|:---:|:---:|:---:|
| **Yin** | *75%* | *75%* | **Yang** |

---

*Appellations  #1 — #10*
**S.** = South  **E.** = East  **W.** = West

|   |   | *R* | *L* |
|---|---|:---:|:---:|
| **1.** Insightful Crane sweeps to the south. | **s.** | ◯ | ⬤ |
| **2.** Secure the right wing. | **s.** | ◯ | ⬤ |
| **3.** Crane spreads his right wing open. | **s.** | ◯ | ⬤ |
| **4.** Secure the left wing. | **s.** | ◯ | ⬤ |
| **5.** Crane spreads his left wing open. | **s.** | ◯ | ⬤ |
| **6.** Powerful bird holds up the sky. | **s.** | ◯ | ⬤ |
| **7.** Advance to release. | **e.** | ◯ | ◑ |
| **8.** Immaculate bird strikes its prey. | **e.** | ◐ | ◯ |
| **9.** Diligent Crane rotates its beak. | **e.** | ◐ | ◯ |
| **10.** Divine bird looks to the heavens. | **e.** | ◯ | ◑ |

*Appellations* **#11 – #20**

S. = *South*  E. = *East*  W. = *West*

| | | *R* | *L* |
|---|---|---|---|
| **11.** Ambitious Crane looks for food. | e. | ◐ | ◐ |
| **12.** Heroic bird stretches his wings. | w. | ◐ | ○ |
| **13.** Uncanny crane stomps his foot. | w. | ◑ | ○ |
| **14.** Fearless bird grabs a fish. | w. | ○ | ◐ |
| **15.** Poignant bird embraces the new day. | w. | ○ | ● |
| **16.** Insightful Crane sweeps to the west. | w. | ○ | ● |
| **17.** Lofty bird goes down under. | e. | ◐ | ○ |
| **18.** Crane spreads his right wing open. | e. | ○ | ● |
| **19.** Angry Crane flaps his wings. | e. | ○ | ● |
| **20.** The agile bird points to the south. | e. | ○ | ● |

# "Closing Movement"

**The Salute:** *A gracious bird salutes the heavens.*

**The Embrace:** *A poignant bird embraces the new day.*

# Resolute Stepping pt. I

*Start out in the ready position, facing south.
As the sun rises in the east, it sets in the west.*

| | | |
|---|---|---|
| ↖ North West | ↑ North | North ↗ East |
| ← West | ↑ ← Centre → ↓ | East → |
| South West ↙ | South ↓ | South East ↘ |

**Left foot = L    R = Right foot**

---

YIN = *Negative*, or   ● / ○   or, *positive* = YANG

In order for one to understand Resolute Stepping, you must first understand chi, or (*life force*). To understand chi, you should understand yin and yang. **Yin & Yang** are the basics of the universe, thus they can be found everywhere. As I understand myself I understand others, as the illness becomes clear to me. Understand the external symptoms, and discover knowledge of the internal in itself.

# The Ready Position pt. I

Face to the south as the sun rises in the east & sets in the west. This allows the warmth of the sun to heat the body. This is done also to give the body a daily amount of sunlight to help produce **Vitamin - D,** that is vital to your bones. For those of you who deal with or suffer from sensitivity to the sun, or **Lupus**, it is advised that these, and the exercises to come be performed inside.

A & Ω

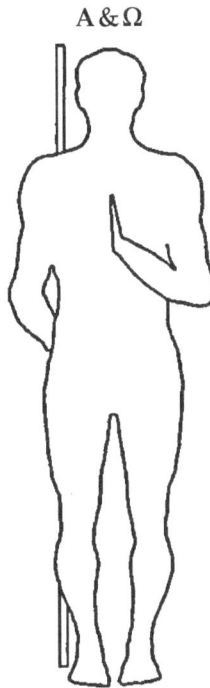

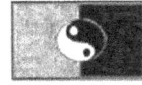

*Right Ft.*      *Left Ft.*

R          L

*yang*        *yin*

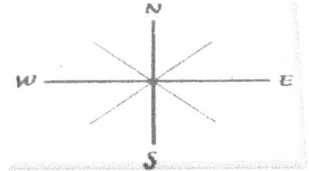

R.  L.        Soft  &  Hard

hen releasing energy, your body should be positioned in such a way, that the sum of the entire body is coordinated into the movement. The flowing process is uninhibited.

**#1** *Express continuity while issuing energy.*

**#2** *There is alertness of the senses, which is unconscious effort.*

**#3** *There is no segregation of movement.*

**#4** *Flawless actions require perpetual motion, which is the proper* ***form & function.***

# Salute the Heavens.

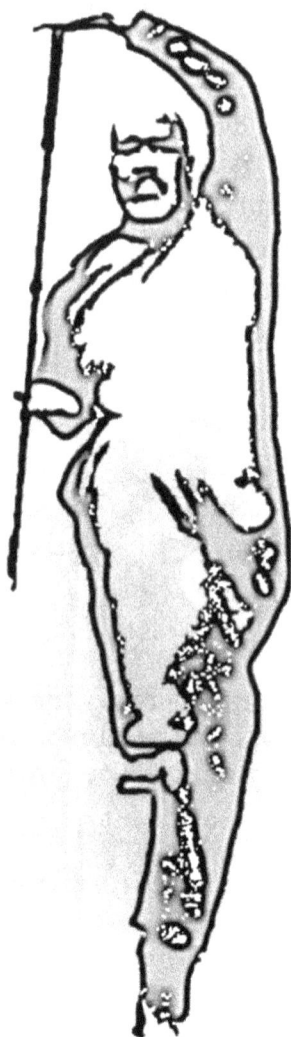

The

月亮

Dark

致敬的天堂，

Yin - The Divine Spear

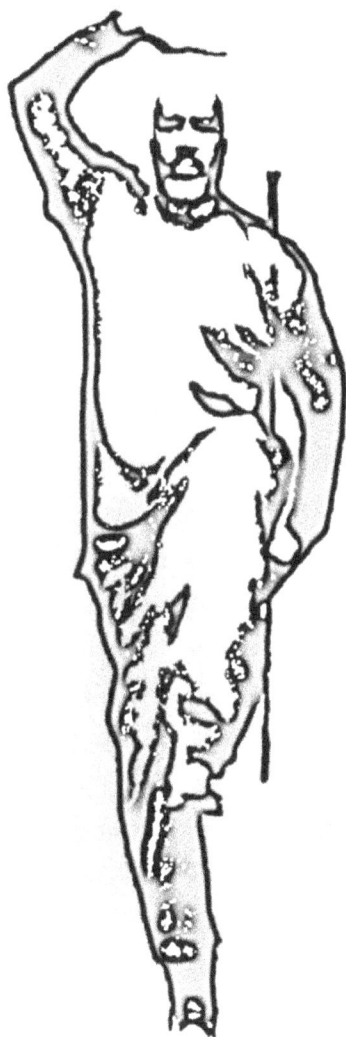

*Embrace the new day.*

迎接新的一天

The 太阳 Light

Yang - The Intrinsic Staff

**1 - 3 S.**

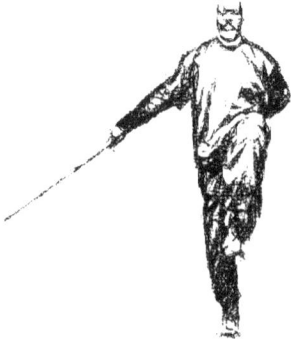

R. L.

**4 - 6 S.**

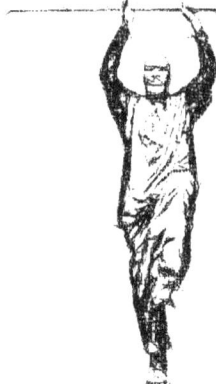

R. L.

**7 E.**

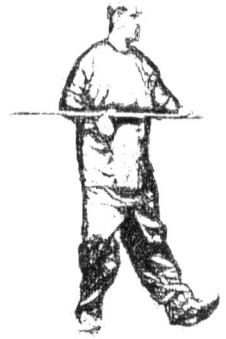

R.          L.

**11 E.**

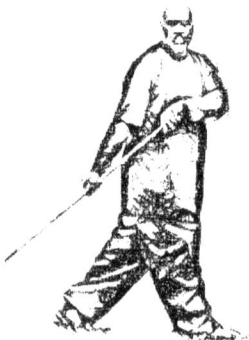

L.          R.

**12 W.**

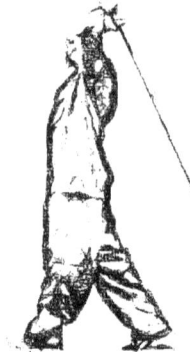

L.          R.

**13 W.**

*Exe. 1-20 using*
**Bamboo Stick**
*48"- 4ft. Long*

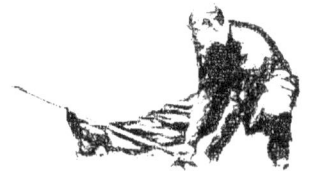

R.                    L.

**17A / W.**

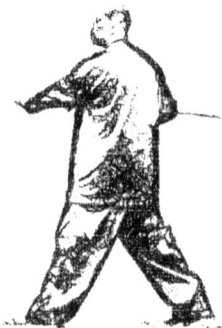

L.          R.

**17B / E.**

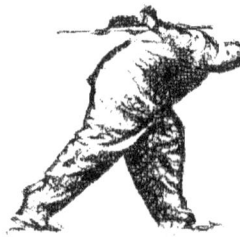

R.          L.

**18A.**

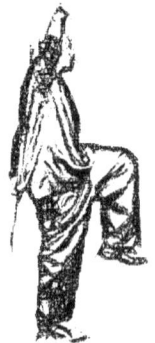

R.     L.

| 8 E. | 9 E. | 10 E. |
|---|---|---|
| 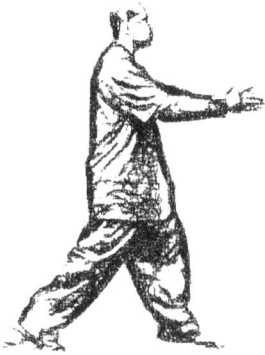 | 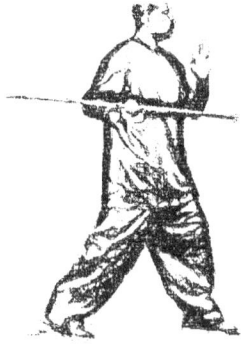 | 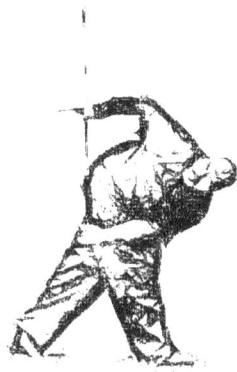 |
| R.          L. | R.          L. | L.          R. |

| 14 W. | 15 W. | 16 W. |
|---|---|---|
| 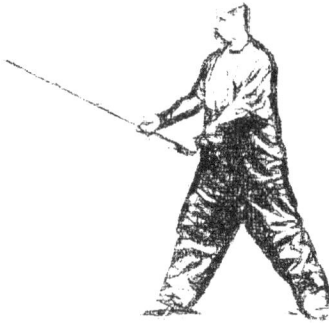 | 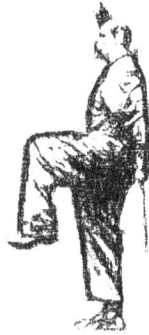 | 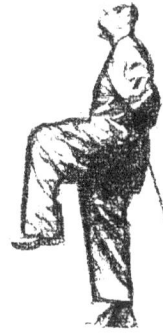 |
| R.          L. | L.          R. | L.          R. |

| 18B / E. | 19 E. | 20 E. |
|---|---|---|
| 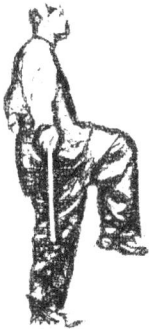 | 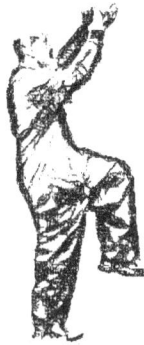 | 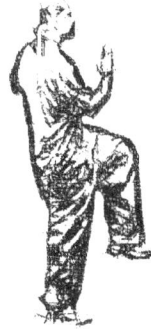 |
| R.          L. | R.          L. | R.          L. |

# Resolute Stepping pt. II

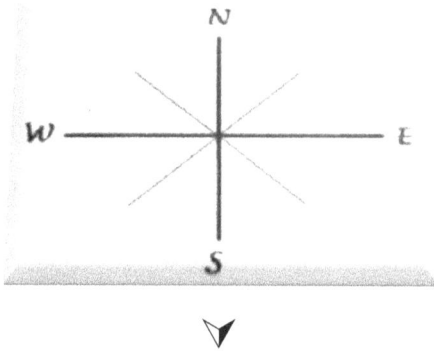

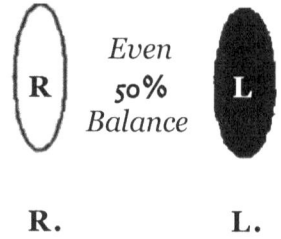

**YANG & YIN**

*Even*
*50%*
*Balance*

R

L

R.    L.

---

●=0%      ◐=TOES      ◑=HEEL      ○=100%
**Yin**     *75%*        *75%*       **Yang**

YIN = *Negative*, or   ● / ○   or, *Positive* = YANG

*Left Foot* = ( *L* )   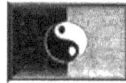   ( *R* ) = *Right Foot*

### Authors Note

As the advance is initiated whether it is left hand lead or right hand lead, its polarity is considered **Yang (creative)**. As the elbow drives the hand forward, its polarity is **Yin**. When you advance or initiate an action, the leading portion of the body would be **Yang**, as the latter half or opposite side would be **Yin**. When any aggressive act is applied to the upper most part of the body, you would change and become empty dispelling the act. The bottom half of your body is **Yang**. Be it mental or physical, any aggressive or negative action of any kind will not penetrate your persona when you exemplify yourself as being empty, and yielding.

For an accurate example, follow along on youtube.
**http://www.youtube.com/weishendo**

# The Ready Position

A & Ω

Upper
Right
Side

Upper
Left
Side

*soft*

*hard*

R.

L.

Tan Tien

*yang*

*yin*

Lower
Right
Side

Lower
Left
Side

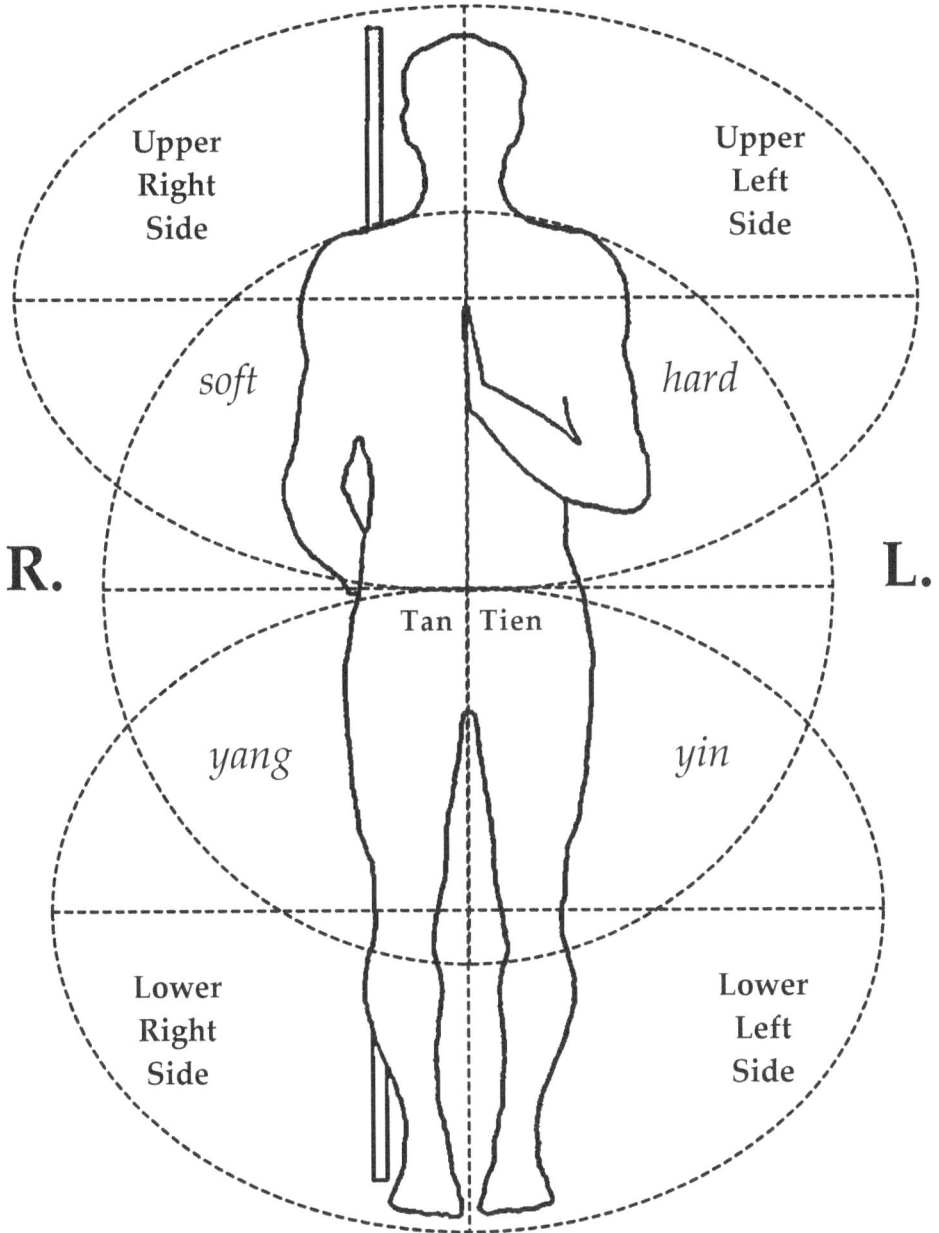

*Face south starting in the ready position.*
*Each diagram coincides with its Appellation.*

# A gracious bird salutes the Heavens.

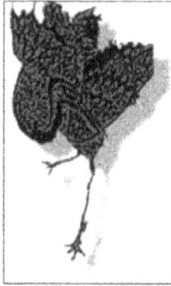

*Facing South*

*YIN*

*Breathe In*

*Expand*

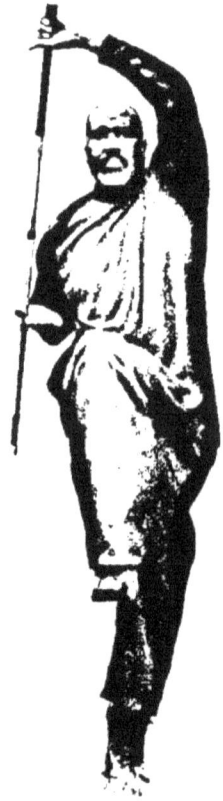

**#1** Starting out in The Ready Position, the right hand comes out holding the staff twirling it one time in a figure eight, **proximal** to the body.

**#2** After this, the right leg is raised with the knee bent at a 90° angle, as the foot is pointing down to the floor. The left hand rises in sync with the right foot, and does a **semi-circle** in a **clock-wise** motion, just above the head to grab the bottom of the staff.

**#3** The final position ends with the right palm facing up in **supination** with the thumb, and **forefinger** holding the centre of the staff, as the tip or top of the staff is pointing down.

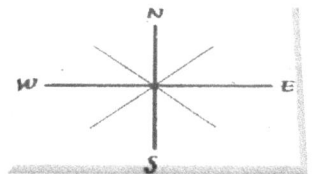

**0%**          **100%**

Right Ft.          Left Ft.

**Yin**     &     **Yang**

# A poignant bird embraces the new day.

*Facing South*

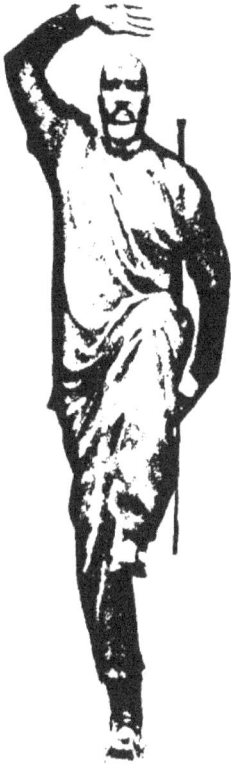

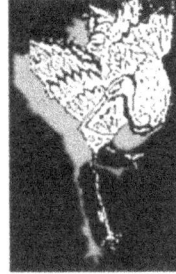

*YANG*

<u>*Breathe Out*</u>

*Contract*

**#1** The right leg drops down, and is followed by the left hand lowering in **proximal** at a ¼ arc, as you hold on to the bottom of the staff.

**#2** As you loosen your grip in the right hand proceed to do another figure eight in **proximal** of the body. Releasing the grip in the left hand, you simultaneously reach out with your left hand and finish the figure eight with the left hand, pulling the staff behind the left side of the body.

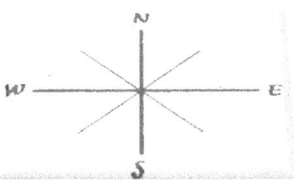

**100%**    **0%**

Right Ft.         Left Ft.

**Yang    &    Yin**

**#3** Raise your right hand above your head in **supination** and in sync with the left leg, as it rises up to a 90° angle bent from the knee with the foot pointing downward. The staffs tip points down.

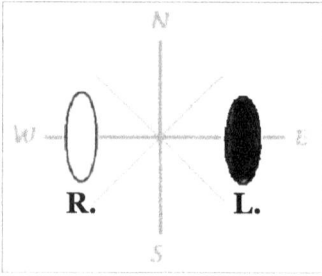

**Face South**

*Insightful Crane sweeps to the south.*

**Segment One**

#1    **Yin** ↓

---

**Face South**

*Secure the right wing.*

**Segment One**

#2    **Yang** ↓

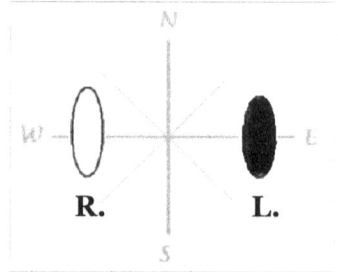

---

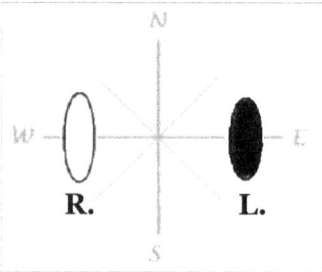

**Face South**

*Crane spreads his right wing open.*

**Segment One**

#3    **Yin** ↓

---

## *A*uthors *N*ote

*As you expand (yin),*
*so must you contract (yang).*
As you do, so must you undo.

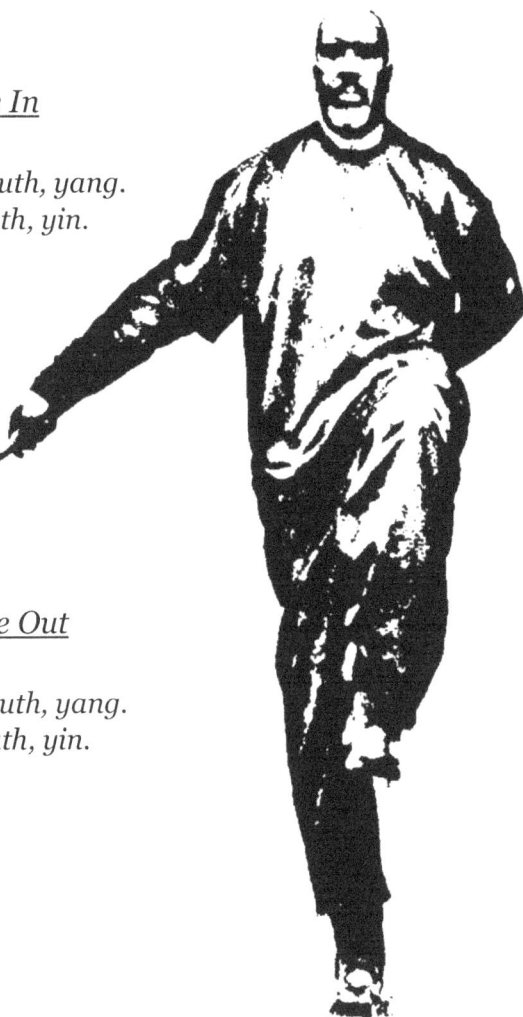

**ℰxa. #1 (** *Resolute Stepping* **)**
**Appellations** *#1 - #3 - <u>Superior Yin</u>*

**#1  <u>Yin</u>** *- <u>Breathe In</u>*

**100%**  Right Ft. *- facing south, yang.*
**0%**  Left Ft. *- facing south, yin.*

**#2  <u>Yang</u>** *- <u>Breathe Out</u>*

**100%**  Right Ft. *- facing south, yang.*
**0%**  Left Ft. *- facing south, yin.*

**#3  <u>Yin</u>** *- <u>Breathe In</u>*

**100%**  Right Ft. *- facing south, yang.*
**0%**  Left Ft. *- facing south, yin.*

*R.      L.*

***yang  &  yin***

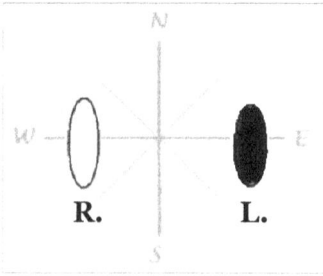

**Face South**

*Secure the left wing.*

**Segment One**

#4      **Yang**    ↓

---

**Face South**

*Crane spreads his left wing open.*

**Segment One**

#5      **Yin**    ↓

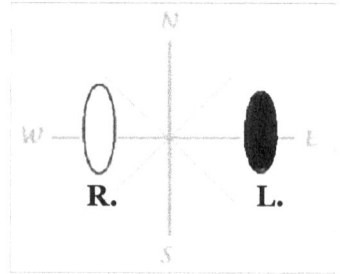

---

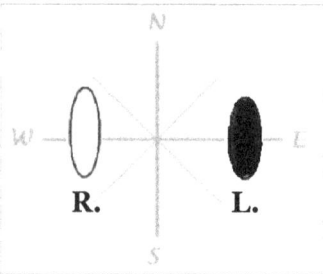

**Face South**

*Powerful bird holds up the sky.*

**Segment One**

#6      **Yang**    ↓

---

## Authors Note

If you have these two things?
#1 Knowledge  #2 Understanding
You have meaning, and insight.

# Exa. #2 ( Resolute Stepping )
## appellations #4 - #6 - Superior Yang

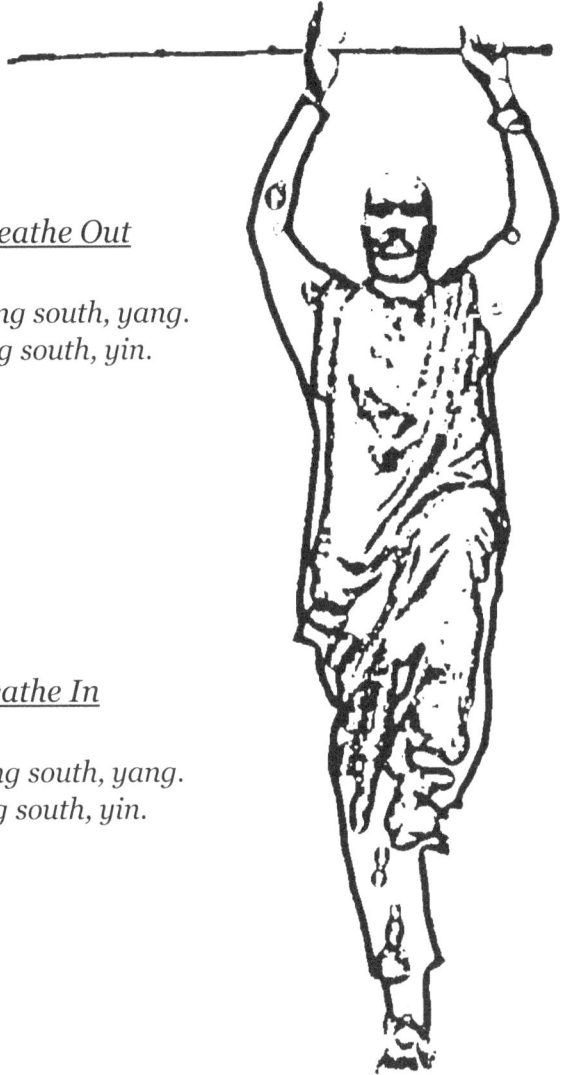

#4  **Yang** - *Breathe Out*

**100%** Right Ft. - *facing south, yang.*
**0%**  Left Ft. - *facing south, yin.*

#5  **Yin** - *Breathe In*

**100%** Right Ft. - *facing south, yang.*
**0%**  Left Ft. - *facing south, yin.*

#6  **Yang** - *Breathe Out*

**100%** Right Ft. - *facing south, yang.*
**0%**  Left Ft. - *facing south, yin.*

R.     L.

**yang & yin**

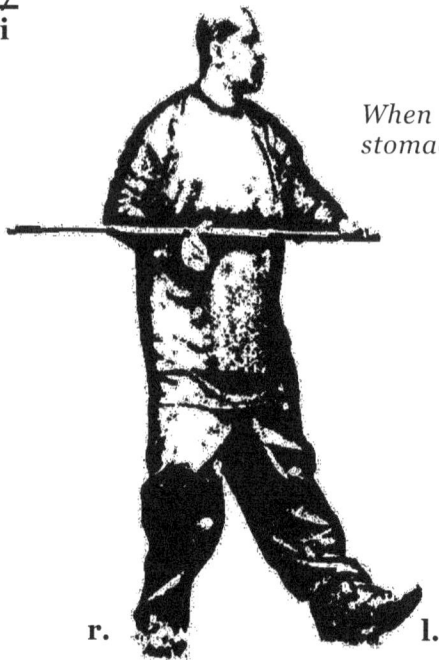

r.          l.

## Yin - *Breathe In*

*When you breathe in it is yin. The stomach expands as you breathe in.*

*Even*
● 50% ○
*Balance*

### YIN = *Negative*

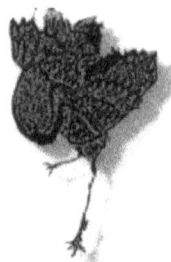

*The Dark*

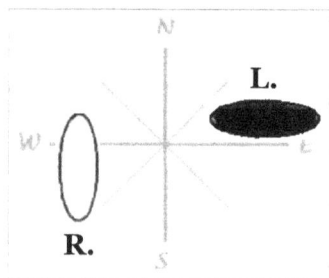

L.

R.

### Face East

*Advance to release.*

**Segment Two**

## Yin          →

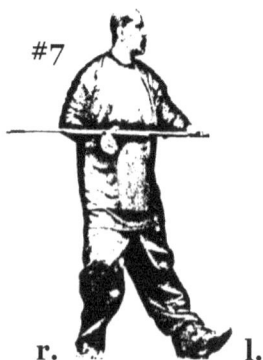

#7

r.          l.

## Yin - *Breathe In*

**80%** Right Foot - *facing south, yang.*
**20%** Left Foot - *facing east, yin.*

## Yang - *Breathe Out*

*When you breath out it is yang. The stomach muscles contracts as you breathe out.*

*Even*
● 50% ○
*Balance*

YANG = *positive*

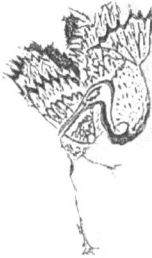

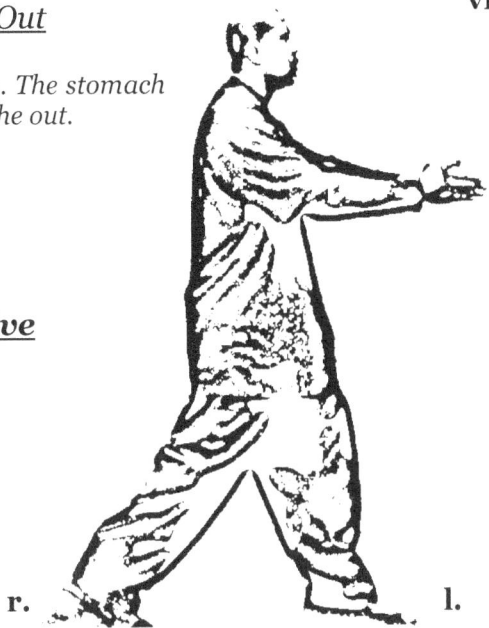

*The light*

r.                                                                  l.

---

### Face East

*Immaculate bird strikes its prey.*

### Segment Two

## Yang    ➔

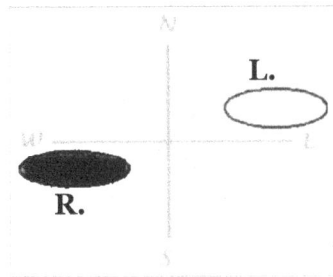

L.

R.

## Yang - *Breathe Out*

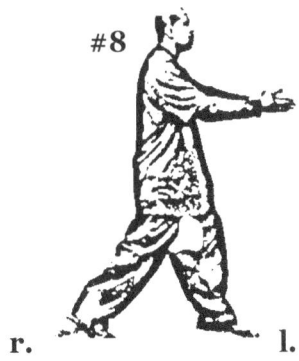

#8

**70%** Right Foot - *facing east, yin.*
**30%** Left Foot - *facing east, yang.*

r.                                                                  l.

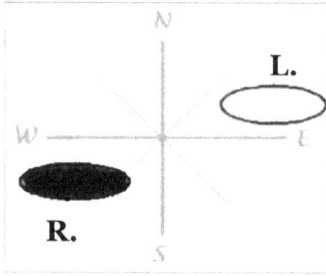

### Face East

*Diligent Crane rotates its beak.*

**Segment Two**

**#9**     **Yin**    →

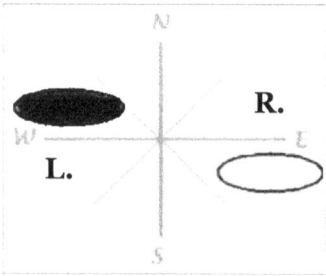

### Face East

*Divine bird looks to the heavens.*

**Segment Two**

**#10**     **Yang**    →

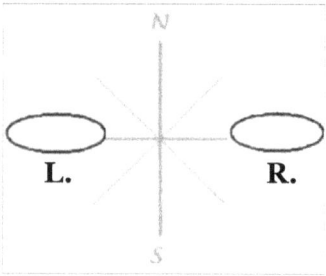

### Face East

*Ambitious Crane looks for food.*

**Segment Two**

**#11**     **Yin**    →

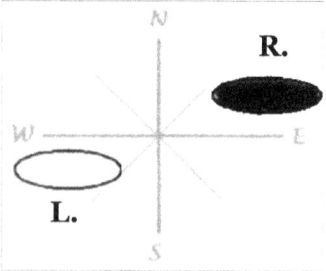

### Face West

*Heroic bird stretches his wings.*

**Segment Three**

**#12**     **Yin**    ←

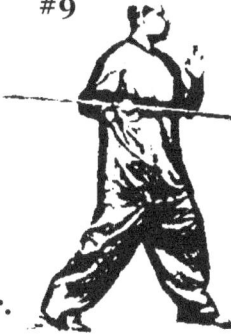

## #9   <u>Yin</u> - *Breathe In*

**50%** Right Foot - *facing east, yin.*
**50%** Left Foot - *facing east, yang.*

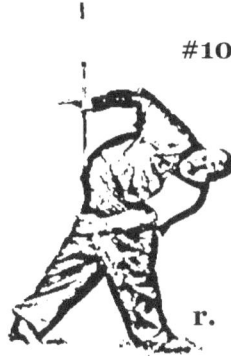

## #10   <u>Yang</u> - *Breathe Out*

**90%** Right Foot - *facing east, yang.*
**10%** Left Foot - *facing east, yin.*

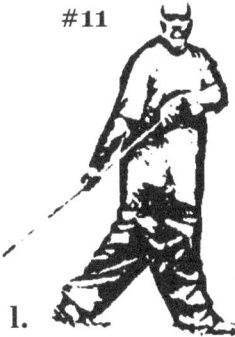

## #11   <u>Yin</u> - *Breathe In*

**50%** Right Foot - *facing east, yang.*
**50%** Left Foot - *facing east, yang.*
*Turn left 180 degrees, face west.*

### Continue to breathe in through exe. #12.

## #12   <u>Yin</u> - *Breathe In*

**30%** Right Foot - *facing west, yin.*
**70%** Left Foot - *facing west, yang.*

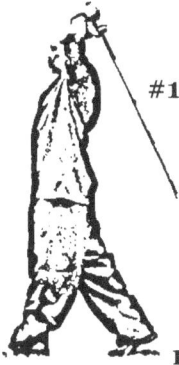

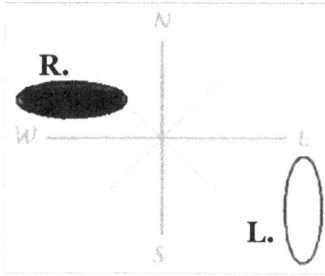

## Face West

*Uncanny Crane, stomps his foot.*

### Segment Three

**#13**    **Yang**    ←

---

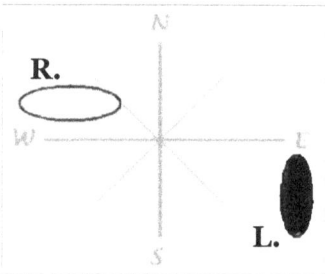

## Face West

*Fearless bird grabs a fish.*

### Segment Three

**#14**    **Yin**    ←

---

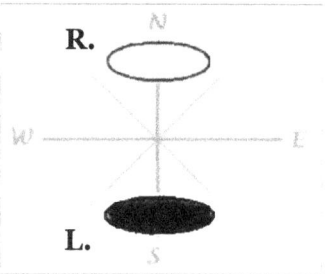

## Face West

*Poignant bird embraces the new day.*

### Segment Three

**#15**    **Yang**    ←

---

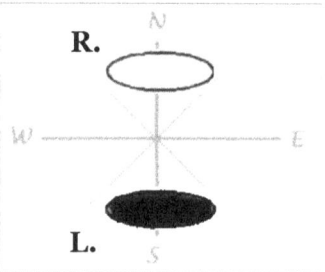

## Face West

*Insightful Crane sweeps to the west.*

### Segment Three

**#16**    **Yin**    ←

#13

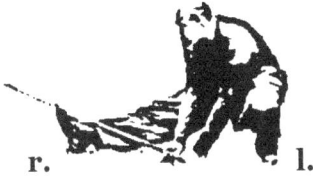

r.          l.

### #13  Yang - *Breathe Out*

**10%** Right Foot - *facing west, yin.*
**90%** Left Foot - *facing south, yang.*

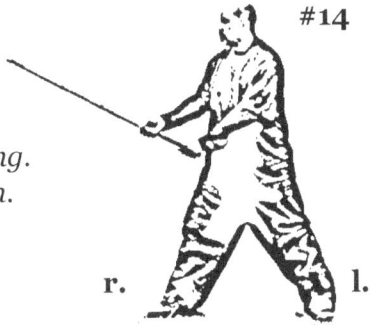

#14

r.          l.

### #14  Yin - *Breathe In*

**50%** Right Foot - *facing west, yang.*
**50%** Left Foot - *facing south, yin.*

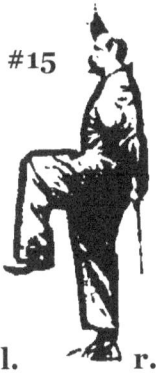

#15

l.      r.

### #15  Yang - *Breathe Out*

**100%** Right Foot - *facing west, yang.*
**0%** Left Foot - *facing west, yin.*

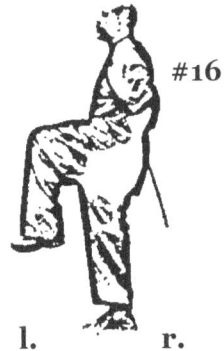

#16

### #16  Yin - *Breathe In*

**100%** Right Foot - *facing west, yang.*
**0%** Left Foot - *facing west, yin.*

l.      r.

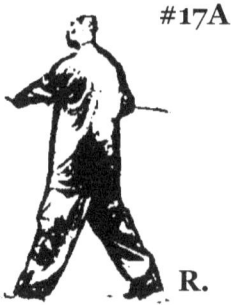

#17A

## #17A  **Yang** - *Breathe Out*
**20%** Right Ft. - *facing west, yang.*
**80%** Left Ft. - *facing west, yin.*
*Turn right 180° degrees, face east.*

### Continue to breathe out until exe. #17B.

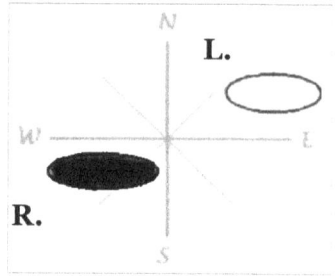

L.

R.

### Face East

*Lofty bird goes down under.*

### Segment Four

## Yin ➔

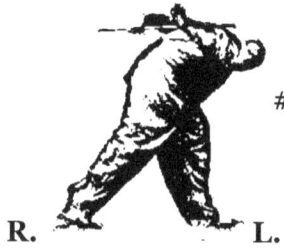

#17B

## #17B  **Yin** - *Breathe in*
**10%** Right Ft. - *facing east, yin.*
**90%** Left Ft. - *facing east, yang.*
*Step forward with the right foot.*

R.

L.

---

## #19  **Yang** - *Breathe Out*

**100%** Right Foot - *facing east, yang.*
**0%** Left Foot - *facing east, yin.*

### Face East

*Angry Crane flaps his wings.*

### Segment Four

## Yang ➔

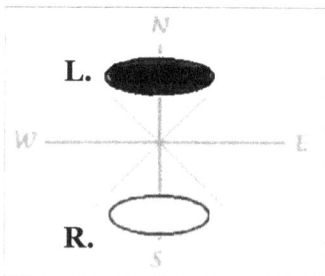

L.

R.

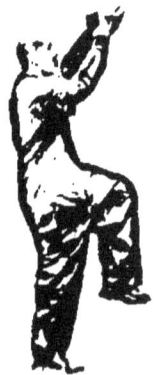

R.     L.

## #18A  Yang - _Breathe Out_
**100%** Right Ft. - _facing east, yang._
**0%** Left Ft. - _facing east, yin._

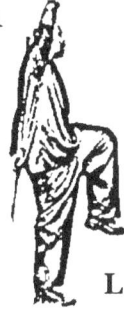

**#18A**

**Continue to breathe out until exe. #18B.**

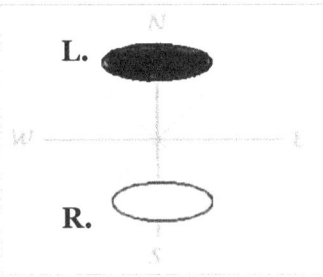

**R.**    **L.**

**Face East**

_Crane spreads his right wing open._

**Segment Four**

**Yin** ➜

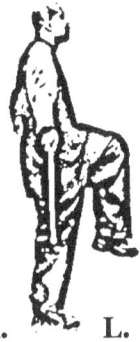

## #18B  Yin - _Breathe In_
**100%** Right Ft. - _facing east, yang._
**0%** Left Ft. - _facing east, yin._

**#18B**

**R.**    **L.**

---

## #20  Yin - _Breathe In_

**100%** Right Foot - _facing east, yang._
**0%** Left Foot - _facing east, yin._

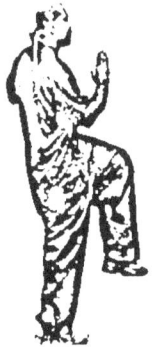

**Face East**

_Agile bird points to the south._

**Segment Four**

**Yin** ➜

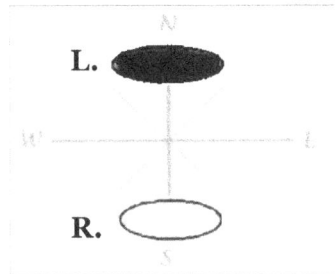

**L.**

**R.**

**R.**    **L.**

# The Ready Position
### A & Ω

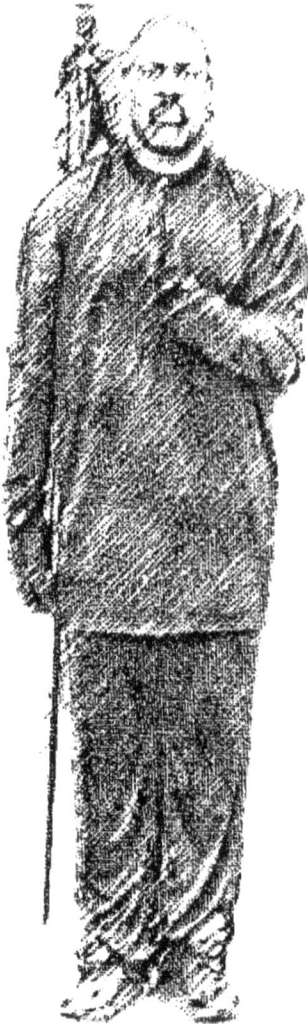 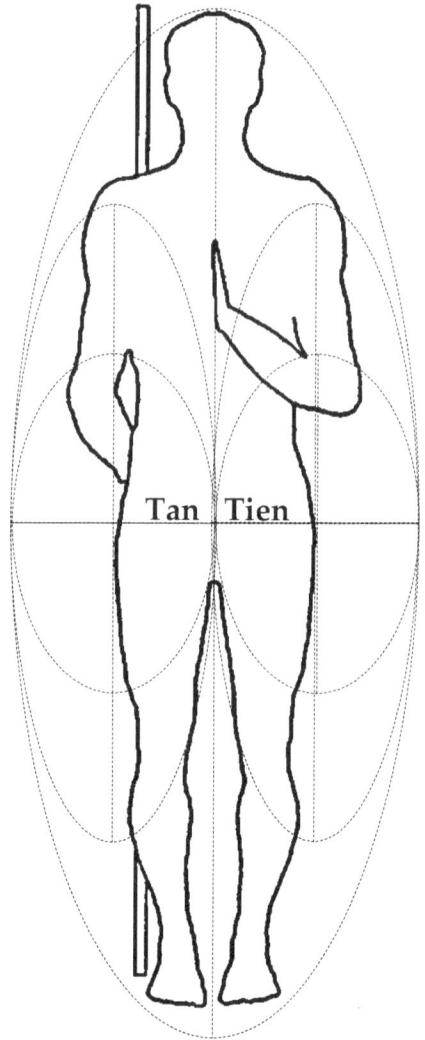

Tan Tien

## *A*uthors *N*ote

*The completion of the exercise ends with you facing to the east. At this point, you can continue to repeat the entire routine again, or stop.* **If you decide to stop, reposition yourself back at,** *The Ready Position* (*Facing South*).

# THE CRANE FORM

**THE SALUTE:** *A gracious bird salutes the heavens.*

**THE EMBRACE:** *A poignant bird embraces the new day.*

---

**Appellations**                                          **Exercise Segment 1.**

## face South

1. Insightful Crane sweeps to the south.
2. Secure the right wing.
3. Crane spreads his right wing open.
4. Secure the left wing.
5. Crane spreads his left wing open.
6. Powerful bird holds up the sky.

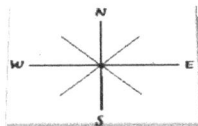

---

**Exercise Segment 2.**

## face East

7. Advance to release.
8. Immaculate bird strikes its prey.
9. Diligent Crane rotates its beak.
10. Divine bird looks 2 the heavens.
11. Ambitious Crane looks for food.

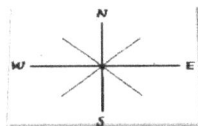

---

**Exercise Segment 3.**

## face West

12. Heroic bird stretches his wings.
13. Uncanny Crane, stomps his foot.
14. Fearless bird grabs a fish.
15. Poignant bird embraces the new day.
16. Insightful Crane sweeps to the west.

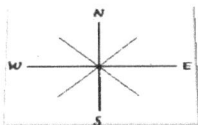

---

**Exercise Segment 4.**

## face East

17. Lofty bird goes down under.
18. Crane spreads his right wing open.
19. Angry Crane flaps his wings.
20. The agile bird points to the south.

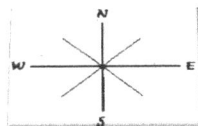

---

# *Chapter #2 Review*

The Crane Form *Simplified Daily Exercise Routine*

Principles

Precepts

---

**Natural Breathing**

**The Human Lungs**

**Meditation**

The Crane Form *Simplified Daily Exercise Routine*

**Resolute Stepping Pt. I**
*The Ready Position* A&Ω

**Resolute Stepping Pt. II**
*The Ready Position* A&Ω

# The Crane Form

*Salute the Heavens,*

*and embrace the new day.*

致敬的天堂，

迎接新的一天。

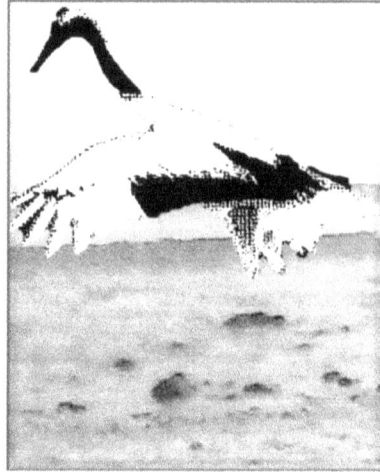

*I*t should be understood by now, that the purpose of any intent is to balance out the execution of the motion. With this being said, our action, or actions are another form of duality. **Yin & Yang** actions are set along a simplistic duality. The following movements to come are an example of the latter. Having done to little or too much will give way to balance. Over extending to engage destroys the form, and its intent. It must be understood that reaching beyond our boundaries will give up our present position at an improper time. (**Relinquishing – vs. – Neutralizing**). Unwanted motion implies a restless spirit. Anticipate the action on a timed or counter stroke. Lead but do not follow. Follow but do not harass. Invite the implied action with non-action. Giving way does not imply defeat. It gives you the opportunity to decrease by adhering to, **The Tao....**

# Chapter 3.

## The Divine Spear
## &
## The Intrinsic Staff

## The Crane Form *Part 2*
## Simplified Daily Exercise Routine

---

## Productive Limits

Feel the moment before it occurs and,
pause the action, stop the action.

Examine the response and,
reactivate the non-active.

The internal awareness of any process is a pausing
action, that is to say, an evaluation of the reactions....

# The Spear (Qiang)

## The King of Long Weapons

Because the spear was generally light, it could be wielded around with quickness and agility. The movements were compared to a dragon. The spear was mainly used for stabbing but could be used for sweeps, slashes, and blocks. All blocking is done with the shaft part of the spear. Considered so versatile a weapon it was given the name, **"The King of Long Weapons."**

The spear that most are familiar with is made of a white wax wood that only grows in Northern China. This wood is favored for its flexible quality. The end is thick but tapers down in thickness, as it gets closer to the tip. The tip is made of forged steel, and is shaped like an arrowhead with a razor sharp edge. The most distinguishing characteristic of the spear is its red tassel that is wrapped at the base of the spearhead. The tassel is used to distract the opponent, and preoccupy him from the spearhead. The tassel also stopped blood from dripping down to the shaft of the spear, as the spear could become very slippery if blood dripped onto the shaft. This also causes the shaft to dry out and become sticky at times, which could affect the sliding techniques of the spear.

### The Length of The Spear
(2 meters) 7 ft. long - to - 13 ft. long (4 meters)

Many Chinese Martial (*military*) Arts required spear training as a necessary part of their daily routine. The overall conditioning that is developed by using the spear is considered an invaluable tool. Many styles have chosen the spear as the first weapon of choice when it comes to alternative training techniques.

# The Staff (Gun)
### The Father of all Weapons

The purpose of the staff is to increase the force delivered, and utilize the length of the weapon. The intrinsic light motion used by the proponent, results in faster forceful motions. This effect made long-range sweeping strikes deadly. The staff can also be lunged forward, thus allowing one to hit from a distance. It is also used for joint-locks, which immobilize the opponent without fatally causing harm. Many techniques, such as kicking and blocking, were combined with the staff when practicing, thus to enhance its effectiveness. There are four basic weapons in the arts. *Of these four, the staff is known as,* **"The Father of All Weapons."**

**1. Gun** - Staff **2. Dao** - Broadsword **3. Qiang** - Spear **4. Jian** - Sword

## The Length of The Staff

**1. Walking Stick** . . . . . . . . . . *½ a person's length, very firm.*

**2. Carrying Stick** . . . . . . . . . . . *¾, or - 0.75" / person's length.*

**3. Rat Tail Staff** . . . . . . . . . . . *Bai - La Wood, same as below.*

**4. Shaolin Staff** . . . . . . . . . . *1 person's length or 5½ to 6½ ft.*

**5. Dragon Staff** . . . . . . . . . *1 ½ a person's length, or 8 to 9 ft.*

The length of the staff is a personal choice, but is roughly 6 ft. **(or 72 in.)** in size. The correct height for a short staff is the height of the practitioner's eyebrow to the floor, with a variance in diameter ranging from 2 inches to ¾ **(or 0.75)** inches. The common staff can be tapered on both ends, tapered to one end, or the same from end to end. This too is a matter of personal choice.

# Spear & Staff

Qiang & Gun (*Chinese; pinyin*) = SPEAR & STAFF

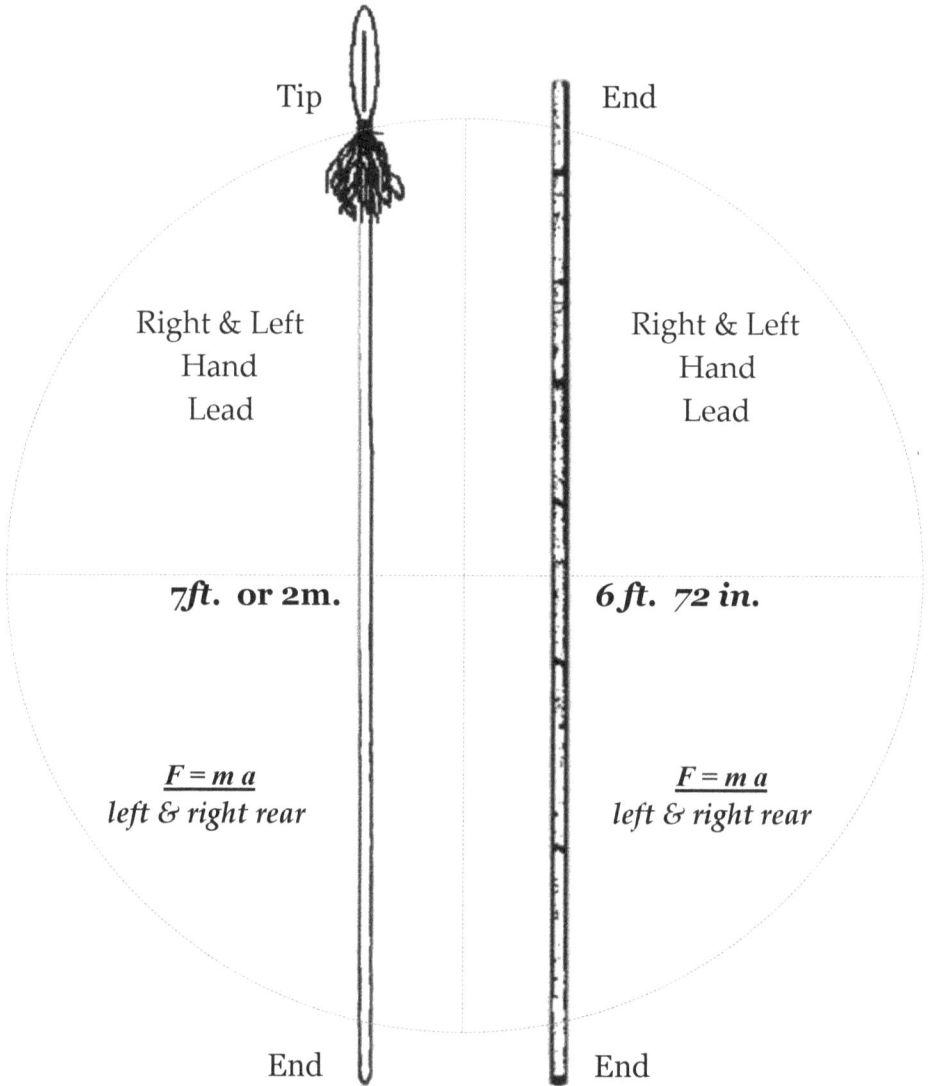

| Tip | End |
|---|---|
| Right & Left Hand Lead | Right & Left Hand Lead |
| **7ft. or 2m.** | **6 ft. 72 in.** |
| $F = m\,a$ left & right rear | $F = m\,a$ left & right rear |
| End | End |

*The sum of the whole, or the equivalence thereof, is the underlying idea of the whole, which is the idea of change. The ongoing continuum, which is* **Constant Change** *- (Yin & Yang).*

# Variations

| Stick | Staff | 3 Sect. | Spear | Kwan Dao | Monks |
|-------|-------|---------|-------|----------|-------|
| Jo | Bo | Staff | | | Spade |

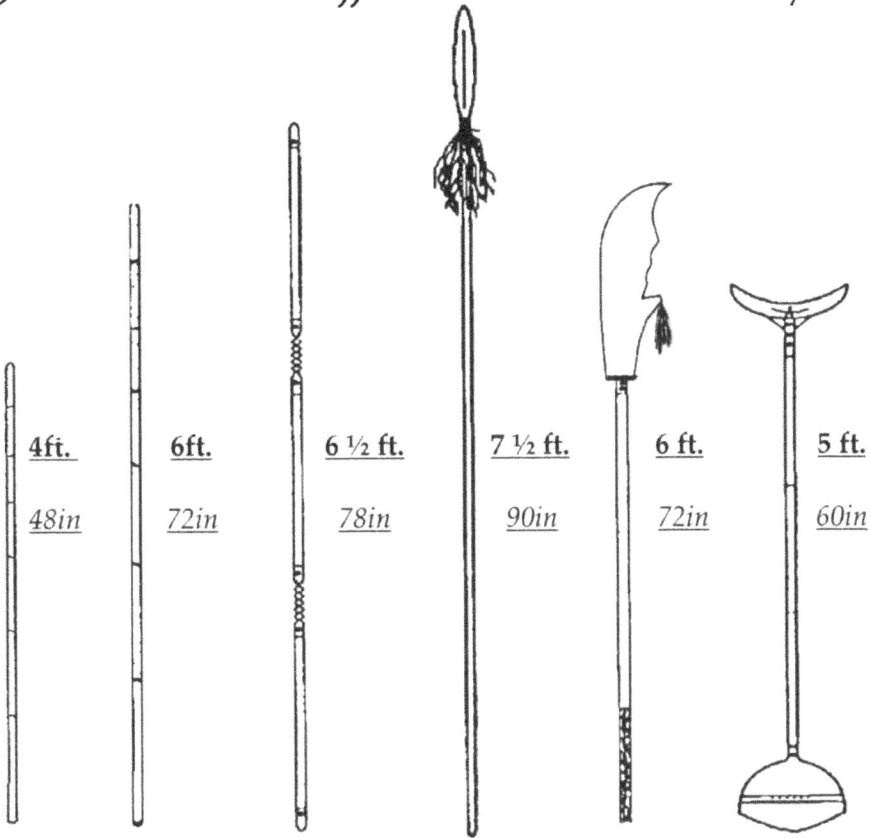

| **4ft.** | **6ft.** | **6 ½ ft.** | **7 ½ ft.** | **6 ft.** | **5 ft.** |
|----------|----------|-------------|-------------|-----------|-----------|
| *48in* | *72in* | *78in* | *90in* | *72in* | *60in* |

## Authors Note

*Shown above are different variations of the spear, and staff. Because of its length, and versatility, the spear is the king of long weapons. The size and length is based on the user and the situation. For our purpose here, we will deal with the practical applications. The basic staff (**Bo**) or stick (**Jo**) will be used throughout the remaining segments in this chapter.*

# The Basic Stance

**A**ssume a basic stance with the right foot forward, but reverse your energy and advance with the lead right hand. As you reverse your energy and advance with the lead right hand, your left hand is held down low to the rear of the staff or spear. In some cases, it is at the very end of the staff. The range and placement will vary according to technique, but the issuing of energy will be the same, be it left or right hand lead. *Ref. pg. 82 - 89*

**Supination** - *is the clockwise or vice versa motion of the forearm and hand as viewed from the proximal end of the limb, or corresponding movement of the feet. The palm of the hand is directed forward, and the thumb moves away from the body.*

**Pronation** - *is the ability to rotate the hand or forearm to bring the palm facing downward or backward. Or, to rotate a joint or part forward and toward the centerline. Counter clockwise motion or vice versa.*

**Proximal** - *is close to or near the point of attachment. A central point, or close to the point of view, which is located toward the centre of the body.*

**Y**ou can train your hands and feet to work together; or in conjunction with each other. When you move, there is a slight moment of weightlessness. This sudden change in balance is not that noticeable at first. But, after hours of practice it becomes ever present that your hands and feet, control equal motion. This uneven effect is an unstable alignment of weight distribution. To know **Kinetic Energy** is to know motion.

$$F = ma$$

*force = momentum & acceleration*

**i.**     **_force_**     *Energy moves through the entire body as a whole, not as a component of the original driving force.*

---

**ii.**     **_Issuing_**     *Advancing involves a relaxed state of mind. The body is calm and silent internally, but externally the appearance is likened to a mountain. You are able to engage, and release the energy within you without effort.*

---

**iii.**     **_form_**     *The natural alive movement of the body can release, and distribute, because the form has followed its natural course.*

---

**iv.**     **_function_**     *The function is applied through a series of motion, which is driven with force, that is issued out of the form.*

---

*The force that you apply is likened, to that of water rushing down a mountain. The limits of such actions can be limitless.*

Yang  Yin

Head

Lead Arm

Lead Hand

r.  l.

$$\frac{S\,t^2 = R}{\infty}$$

$F = m\,a$

Lead Leg  Rear Leg

R.  L.

Yang  Yin

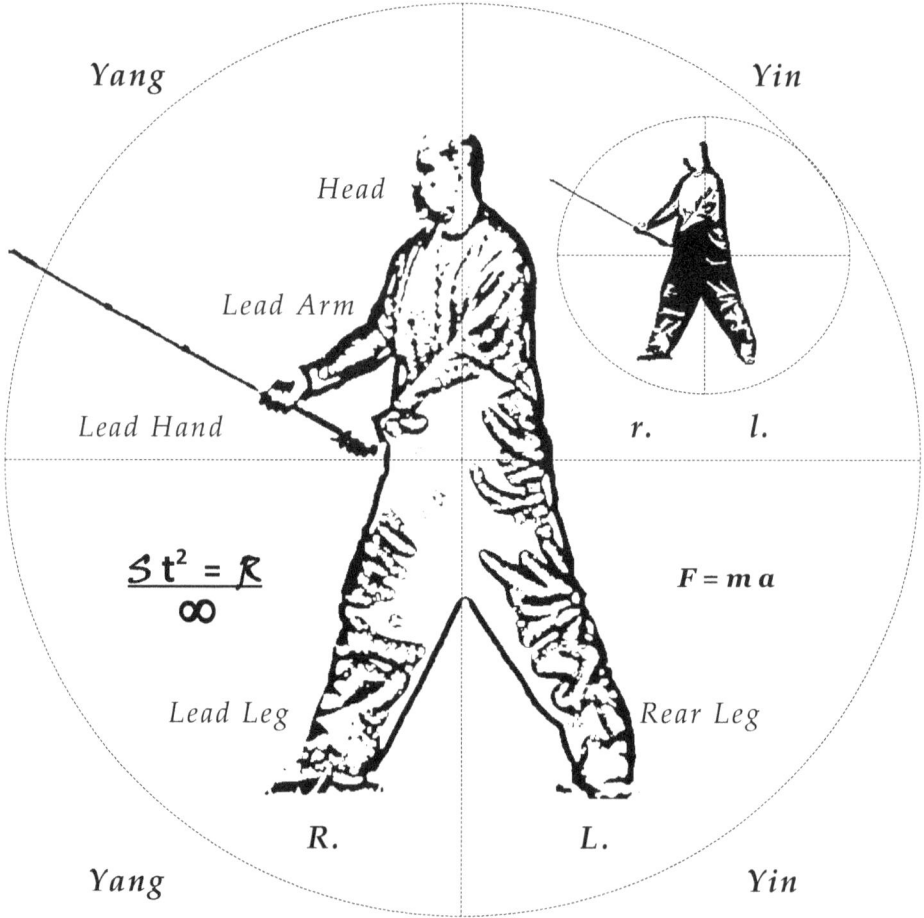

**#1** *You must centralize to a specific space, time, and reality, where your actions are those of the purest. Reaching but not over extending to localize. The Purest establishes his diversion, which is his ability to be centered, by applying division.*

**#2** *In the process of measuring, you should be aware of the area, and the amount of effort it takes to maneuver from one space to another. Survey as a whole, and not as a segregated piece.*

*exa. #1  Basic Stance*

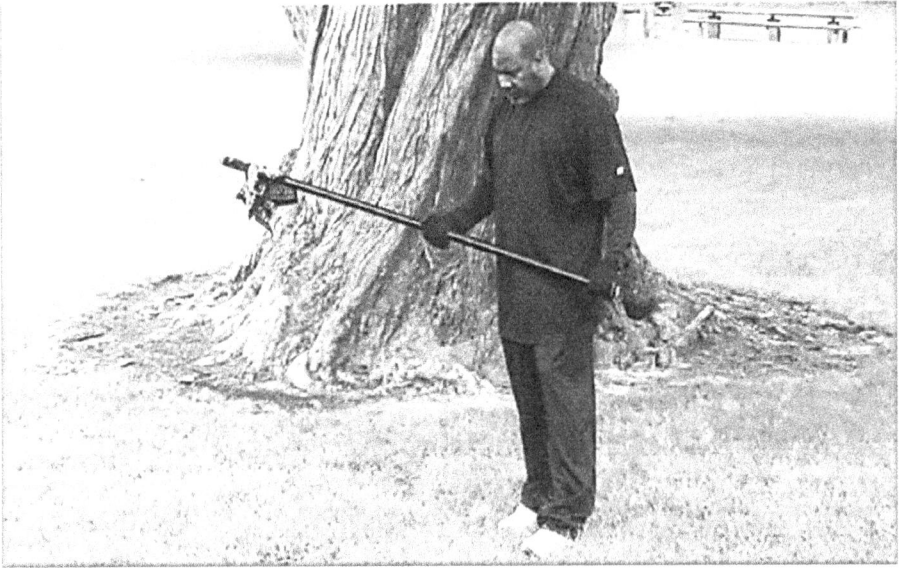

(*Make use of your* **space** {S}, *and occupy your* **time** {t²}, *of which you are now in control of; while being* **realistic** {R}, *in execution*).

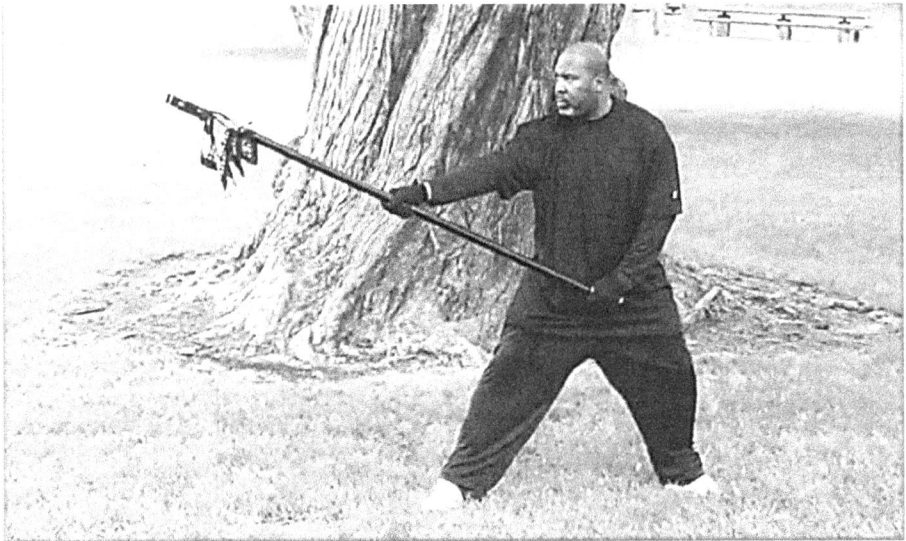

*exa. #2  Basic Stance*

# 1. Throughout this text the basic precept, is that of change.

*The principles of change tell us that, we should*
*be able to calculate in regards to the effort given.*

*The positive, and negative polarities of the body,*
*must be in alignment to maintain balance.*

*This distinction exist in all that is applied in **space**, and*
***time**, while being **realistic**. Such is **The Tao of Wu Wei.***

*Change is fundamentally constructed from non-change,*
*which is relative to... (Non - action a.k.a. **Wu - Wei**).*

It is such an act that the timing and judging of distance is achieved in an instant. An exact placement of the hands and feet appears to be inadequate to the untrained eye. To devise an economical means of positioning the hands, and feet, you must understand, **The 3 Precepts of WEISHENDO.** *(For an accurate description read, "The Principles & Philosophy of WEISHENDO")*

$$a + b = c$$

| **Measurement** | + | **Interception** | = | **Penetration** |
|:---:|:---:|:---:|:---:|:---:|
| Ch'ang | | Chieh | | Ch'uan |

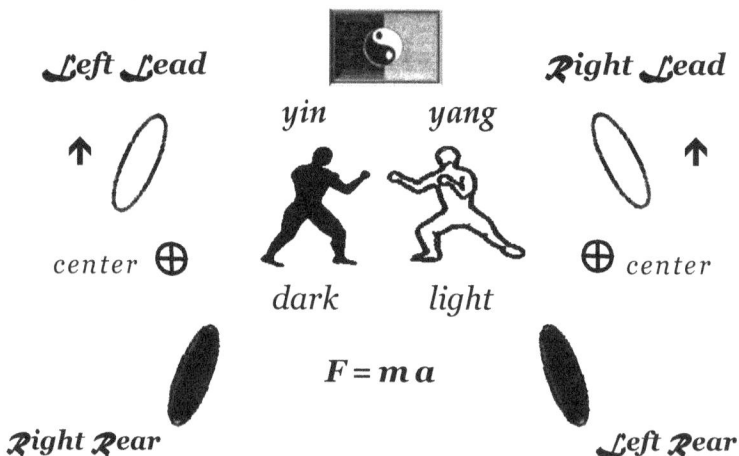

**Left Lead**                    **Right Lead**

yin          yang

center ⊕                    ⊕ center

dark          light

$$F = m\,a$$

**Right Rear**                    **Left Rear**

## 2. Firmness is concealed in softness, and vice - versa.

*(The concept of change is based on two basic but very complex principles.* $\dfrac{\textbf{Light}}{Yang}$ **+** $\dfrac{\textbf{Dark}}{Yin}$ *It is the foundation of which change is built upon. That which can bring about alternation in virtue).* **=** **Efflorescence of Change.**

---

## The Footwork of Yin & Yang
### *Efflorescence of Change*

$F = ma$ - ($F$ = force) ($m$ = momentum) ($a$ = acceleration)

### *Advanced Lead*

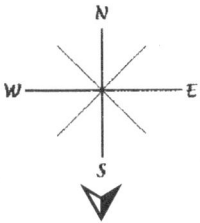

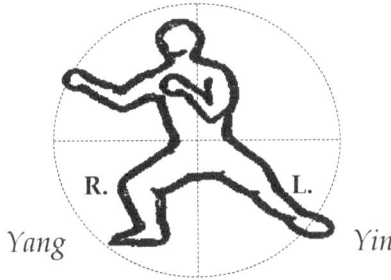

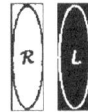

| | | | |
|---|---|---|---|
| yang ⬭ soft<br>**light** | TOE | HEEL | yin ⬮ hard<br>**dark** |
| 75% | 50% | 25% | 0% |

## 3. The methodical process evolves around residual motions.

*For the purest, to lose the force of momentum while in the chain of events means that he has lost the advantage. To ascertain* **THE FLOW.** *A continuum of what is, must be sustained for an optimal amount of time.*

### 1. Reliability        2. Simplicity        3. Practicality

*Having order to your methods gives them organization. You cannot apply any form of penetration, without order.*

**A.** Redirect the effect...
**B.** Absorb the intent...
**C.** You must co-exist, with any force given to your cause.
**D.** Not acting, as a means of acting, to efface momentum.

*By using the latter actions, you can double, or, quadruple your own non-action, with unorthodox effort.*

#1 You must complement every advance with a greeting or salutation. The action you make is a question that is a *stimulus.*

**STIMULUS**
*yang*

#2 You must compliment every retreat with a closing remark. The action you make is an answer to the *response.*

**RESPONSE**
*yin*

#3 Pausing is done out of divisive intent. Having a balance in your *pausing.*

**PAUSING**

## 4. Action is a combined effort of, the totality of oneness.

$$\frac{action}{a\,+\,b\,=\,c} \quad + \quad \frac{reaction}{F\,=\,ma} \quad = \quad \frac{S\,t^2\,=\,R}{\infty}$$

There is a physical and mental state in your execution.
In the methodical process, you understand the principles of,

(**Oneness** - <u>singularity</u>).

---

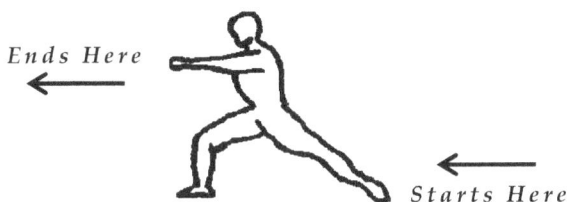

*Ends Here* ←

← *Starts Here*

To properly execute the latter,
you must thoroughly understand,

**Kinetic Energy.**

---

## There is no fixated significance,
## other than this well-known fact.

*We change, in a manner of never showing signs of becoming stagnant.*

Furthermore, we alternate so, that we bring about change. We stimulate so, that we maintain a continuum of constant change. Thus change over a period involves the ability to reproduce an action, which is endless. When we evaluate this changing process, and how relative it is to being infinite we begin to fathom the underlying principle of, **Constant Change.**

# The Five Elements   (*Wu = 5 / Hsing = elements*)

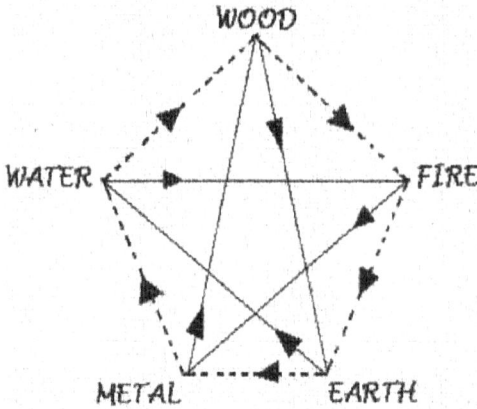

## Wu - Hsing

### 5 - Elements

Water - - - - - - - - - - - - - - - Fire

Fire - - - - - - - - - - - - - - - -Earth

Earth - - - - - - - - - - - - - -Metal

Metal - - - - - - - - - - - - - Water

Water - - - - - - - - - - - - - Wood

*As you study the movements, you must allow yourself time to recover after each segment. Study your momentum and repose long enough to make a second intent. Assess and renew your actions, without any considerable pausing. Such efforts are developments, to the* **productive limits** *of the flow. By having perceptive forethought, you give infinite incite to the way. To be progressive in our process we must understand what is meant by* **productive limits.** *Your actions take on the adaptive property of water.* **(One of the five natural elements).**

To put such methods into play involves the process of **releasing energy** at the opportune time, whereas **issuing energy** requires the stamina to maintain the action. **Residual motion** is the key element. The depths of our movement are along the lengths of control we possess during the intent. The time that is involved in releasing the internal spirit, and the external will of our soul, should be done with maximum effort and minimal pausing.

We end, only to begin as new.
Deep within, is the secret?

---

**Once you have been given a form, you have a structure.**

*(This means your offensive momentum has been constructed into a*

*defensive fixation. You should never allow the opponent to mold or*

*shape you in such a way, that you take on a defensive form or shape).*

**Have a defense, without being defensive.**

←     *or*     →

|           | WOOD            | FIRE           | EARTH     | METAL           | WATER     |
|-----------|-----------------|----------------|-----------|-----------------|-----------|
| TAI CHI   | RETREAT         | GAZE RT.       | CENTRAL   | ADVANCE         | LOOK LT.  |
| DIRECTION | EAST            | SOUTH          | CENTER    | WEST            | NORTH     |
| SEASON    | SPRING          | SUMMER         | LATE SUM. | AUTUMN          | WINTER    |
| YIN       | LIVER           | HEART          | SPLEEN    | LUNG            | KIDNEY    |
| YANG      | GALL BLADDER    | SMALL INTEST.  | STOMACH   | LARGE INTEST.   | BLADDER   |

↑ or ↓

This form of construction, should lead to deconstruction.

# The Four Corners

## Advancing

When there is a chance to advance or move forward, do so without haste. If there is nothing to prohibit your advance, then you can proceed. The opportunity is missed, if you do not execute at the proper time. But alas, if done in time it can be achieved...

## Retreating

When there is a chance to retreat or move backwards, it can quickly change to an advance. To avoid the insubstantial is the way of **THE TAO.** You must strive to seek emptiness. When you are empty, **(yin....)** the execution will be shallow...

## Moving Right

When moving to the right or neutralizing from the right, the true intent comes from the left. To gain an adequate position you must change all advancing, and move to an appropriate position. There can be no second guessing in this method...

## Moving Left

When moving left or neutralizing from the left, it is wise to follow with the right. Everything moves as one. Hands, feet, knees, elbows, waist, head, shoulders, are all one accord. This will leave little for the opponent to distinguish from, thus he will find nothing. **(YIN)**

## Advancing - yang

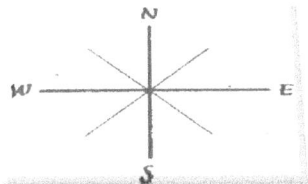

**Yang**       **Yin**

r.            l.

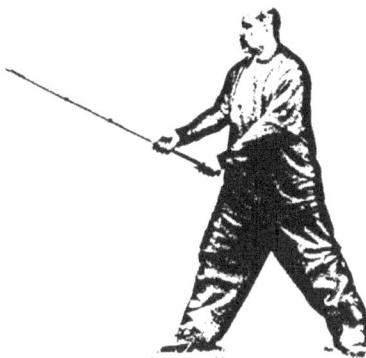

### Retreating - yin

r.     l.

---

**Moving Right**

←

Lt. Ft.

Rt. Ft.

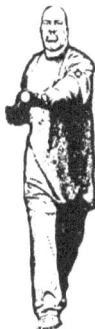

Right
←

Facing South

---

**Moving Left**

→

Lt. Ft.

Rt. Ft.

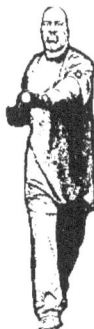

Left
→

Facing South

# The Shuffle

The forward and backward shuffle can be done with short steps in a consecutive motion, to control and maintain balance.

**1.** *From this position, you can quickly shift your body to numerous positions. Because of the shuffle, there is no crossing of feet to achieve another angle. The motion is steady and non-prohibitive. (**There are exceptions to this**).*

**2.** *You can advance and withdraw yourself from one position. When there is freedom of movement without restrain, there is no need to acquire numerous positions?* **Simple & Direct.** (***There are exceptions to this***).

*I*t is important for you to remember, stay light and agile on your feet. It should feel as if you are suspended from a string like a puppet. Footwork is the cornerstone of technique. You must associate to that which will give optimal assimilation of the latter.

# The Side Step

*T*he art of moving left or right is achieved through the constant practice of positioning. It is a safe and effective maneuver, which can create openings for a successful advance. As you move the first step should be in the direction you are about to move. Your body should move first, leaning to the left or right. Execute with precision and tact.

**Authors Note** The latter examples explain movement to a favorable position with the singular purpose on economy of motion, and simplicity in mind. But for the development of **The Crane Form** in the following segments, adhere to the steps.

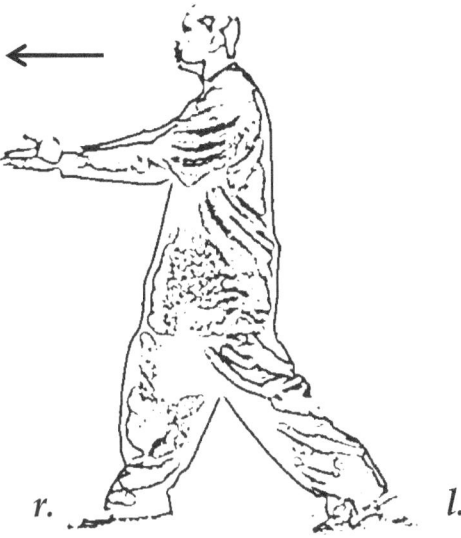

**Right Ft. Lead**

⬭ Right Foot

⬬ Left Foot

*light*

*soft*

**Yang**

r.   l.

---

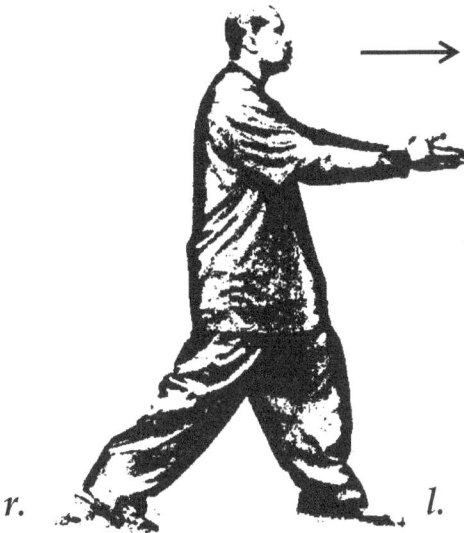

**Left Ft. Lead**

Left Foot ⬭

Right Foot ⬬

*dark*

*hard*

**Yin**

r.   l.

*Co - existence of oneness is the continuum of what is.
Associate to that which will give optimal assimilation.*

## Definition #1

**SPEED** (noun) **- can be defined as the rate of motion or velocity of the body, or any one of its parts.** *Reaction time, which is another component of speed, can be defined as the length of time it takes to respond to any type of stimulus. Any effort to develop speed must concentrate on the type of speed to be developed, be it total body, and limb acceleration, or all out total, and maximal velocity. The execution of speed is generated to the area being developed. The effort is concentrated on the specific body part. The training program must be carefully selected to concentrate on those areas that are important to the user. **Biomechanics** play a very large role in the determination of speed, and the ability to increase it.*

## Definition #2

**AGILITY** (noun) **- can be defined as the maneuverability of the individual.** *The ability to shift to the direction of movement very rapidly; or to move in a specific direction without any loss of balance or sense of position. An overall combination of speed, strength, quick reactions, balance, and coordination, which can be applied to the body as a whole, or to a specific body part, such as the hands or feet.*

# Intangible Motion

*Administer your intent without delayed or stagnant thought.*
*Once the course of action has been determined, apply it.*

*Your follow through or follow up of the second attempt,*
*has already been set in motion due to its continuity.*

---

*Spontaneous action is the equivalence of surprise intent.*
*The intention has been made without **aforemention.***

## 1. *Initial Intention*
## 2. *Renewed Intention*

*The latter was applied within the blink of an eye,*
*catching the opponent distracted, for a brief moment in time.*
*In short, your motion is very elusive, and vague.*

**a + b = c**

> ***Spontaneous Action***
>
> **+** ***Surprise Intent***
>
> **= *Intangible Motion***

## Authors Note

When the slightest pause in execution is detected,
we must manage to ascertain the minuscule possibility of,
flowing, and moving with the fluctuations of **Yin & Yang Principles.**

# Spear (*Qiang*)  Staff (*Gun*)

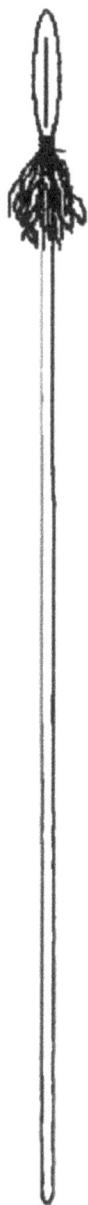

**The Night**
黑 夜
*dark*

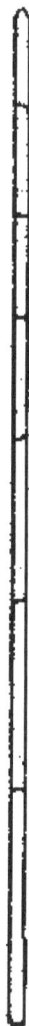

**The Day**
白 天
*light*

*Wax Wood 90in. - 7½ ft.  /  Bamboo 72in. - 6ft.*

# The Crane Form
*The Night,* 黑 夜。 *&* *The Day,* 白 天。

神矛内在工作人员

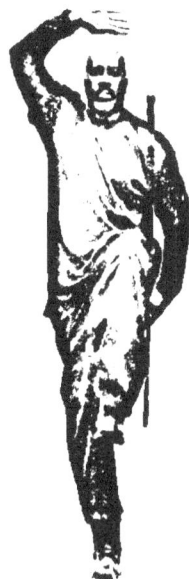

*Divine Spear & Intrinsic Staff*
# WEISHENDO

**_THE SALUTE:_** *A gracious bird salutes the heavens.*

**_THE EMBRACE:_** *A poignant bird embraces the new day.*

---

### *Appellations*

### *Face South*

*Exercise Segment 1.*

1. Insightful Crane sweeps to the south.
2. Secure the right wing.
3. Crane spreads his right wing open.
4. Secure the left wing.
5. Crane spreads his left wing open.
6. Powerful bird holds up the sky.

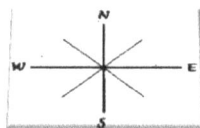

---

*Exercise Segment 2.*

### *Face East*

7. Advance to release.
8. Immaculate bird strikes its prey.
9. Diligent Crane rotates its beak.
10. Divine bird looks 2 the heavens.
11. Ambitious Crane looks for food.

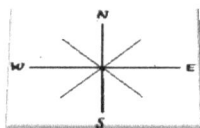

---

*Exercise Segment 3.*

### *Face West*

12. Heroic bird stretches his wings.
13. Uncanny Crane, stomps his foot.
14. Fearless bird grabs a fish.
15. Poignant bird embraces the new day.
16. Insightful Crane sweeps to the west.

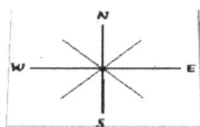

---

*Exercise Segment 4.*

### *Face East*

17. Lofty bird goes down under.
18. Crane spreads his right wing open.
19. Angry Crane flaps his wings.
20. The agile bird points to the south.

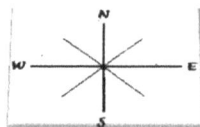

---

*For an accurate example, follow along on youtube.*
http://www.youtube.com/weishendo

# The Ready Position pt.II

*Refer back to the Natural Breathing Chart on pg. 42.*
*Breathe in and out naturally, through each exercise segment.*

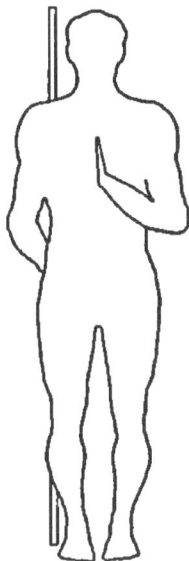

A&Ω

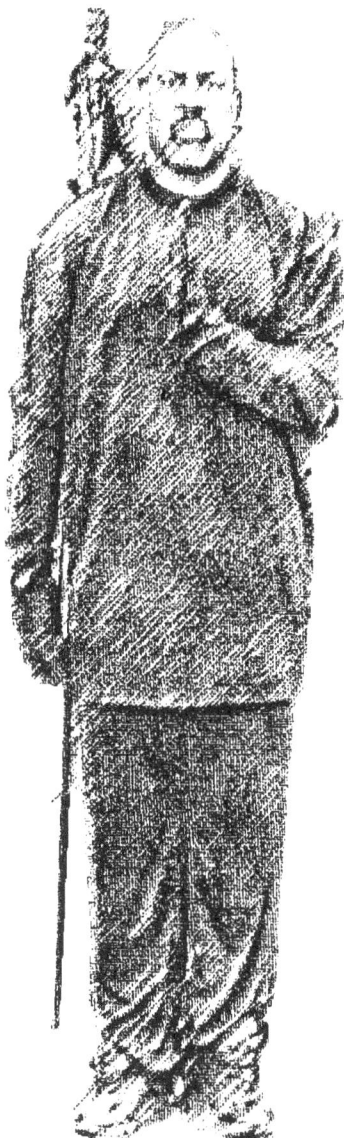

Right ft.    Left ft.

yang       yin

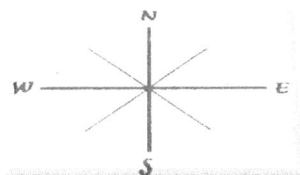

*Face south starting in the ready position.*
*Each diagram coincides with its Appellation.*

# A gracious bird salutes the Heavens.

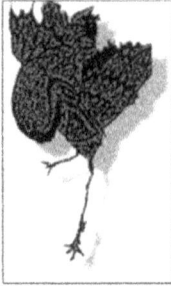

*YIN*

*Breathe In*

*Expand*

**#1** Starting out in The Ready Position, the right hand comes out holding the staff twirling it one time in a figure eight, **proximal** to the body.

**#2** After this, the right leg is raised with the knee bent at a 90° angle, as the foot is pointing down to the floor. The left hand rises in sync with the right foot, and does a **semi-circle** in a **clock-wise** motion, just above the head to grab the bottom of the staff.

**#3** The final position ends with the right palm facing up in **supination** with the thumb, and **forefinger** holding the centre of the staff, as the tip or top of the staff is pointing down.

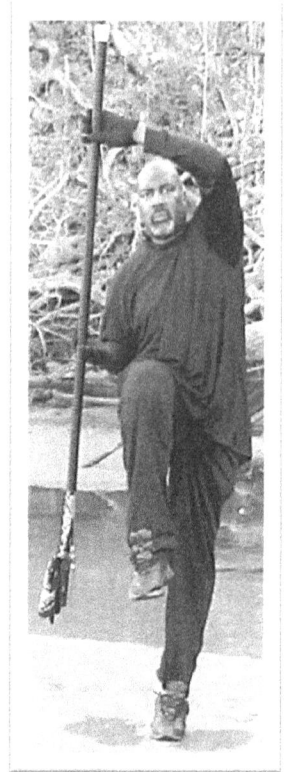

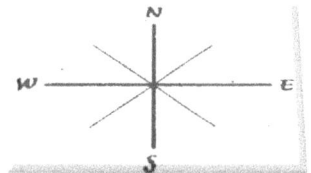

0%                    100%

Right Ft.              Left Ft.

**Yin    &    Yang**

# A poignant bird embraces the new day.

*YANG*

<u>*Breathe Out*</u>

*Contract*

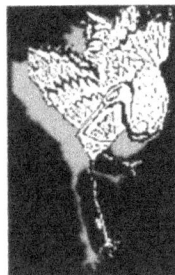

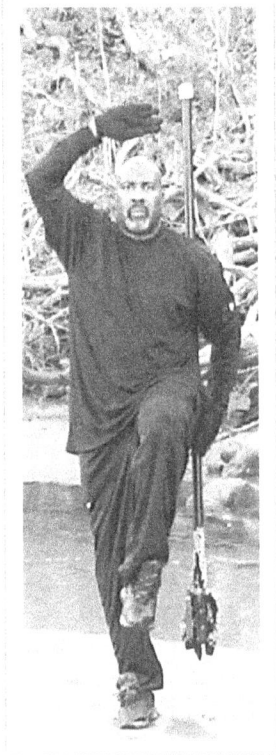

**#1** The right leg drops down, and is followed by the left hand lowering in **proximal** at a ¼ arc, as you hold on to the bottom of the staff.

**#2** As you loosen your grip in the right hand proceed to do another figure eight in **proximal** of the body. Releasing the grip in the right hand, you simultaneously reach out with your left hand and finish the figure eight with the left hand, pulling the staff behind the left side of the body.

**#3** Raise your right hand above your head in **supination** and in sync with the left leg, as it rises up to a 90° angle bent from the knee with the foot pointing downward. The staffs tip points down.

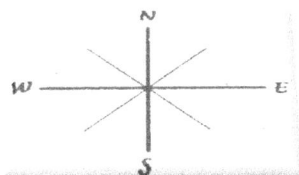

**100%**　　　　**0%**

Right Ft.　　　Left Ft.

**Yang**　**&**　**Yin**

# Exercise Segment – One

**#1 Insightful Crane sweeps to the south** - Engage the right hand bringing it behind your back, as you grab the staff and sweep it around from the north to the south. The tip of the staff should be pointing down towards the ground at a 45° angle. (*The left hand is placed firmly behind the small of the back with your fingers spread open*).

**#2 Secure the right wing** - As the staff comes up in a clock-wise motion **proximal** to the body, the right side of the body has been secured.

**#3 Crane spreads his right wing open** - Continuing with the flow of energy, the right hand raises the staff up from the **proximal** position, lifting it above the head in a circular motion.

**#4 Secure the left wing -** The left hand comes from behind the back to secure the left side in a counter clock-wise motion, **proximal** to the body. The left side of the body has been secured.

**#5 Crane spreads his left wing open** - Continuing with the flow of energy, the left hand rises up from the **proximal** position, twirling the staff above the head in a counter clock-wise motion with the right hand.

**#6 Powerful bird holds up the sky** - The exercise ends with both hands suspended in the air twirling the staff above the head in a counter clock-wise motion, as the left leg is held at a 90° angle. The left foot is pointing down.

*Your weight throughout Exercise Segment - One, is on the right leg.*

## Appellation #1 - #3

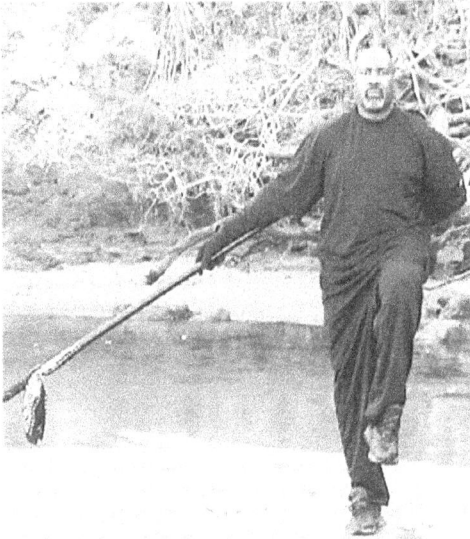

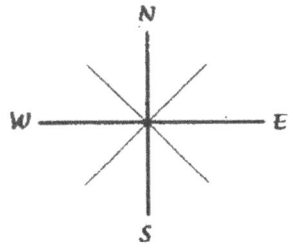

**Right Ft.**    **Left Ft.**

## Appellation #4 - #6

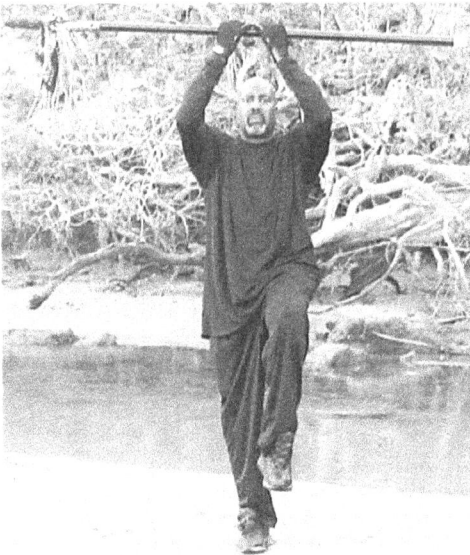

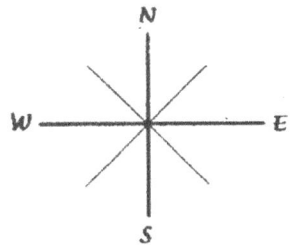

**Right Ft.**    **Left Ft.**

# Exercise Segment – Two

**#7 Advance 2 Release** - From the south position, you rotate 90° to the east from the waist. As the left leg lowers, you touch heel to toe, with the left foot pointing east. The right foot points to the south. Simultaneously bringing the staff across the body, your left hand grips the bottom of the staff, as your right hand grabs the center of the staff.

**#8 Immaculate bird strikes its prey** - The heel of the right foot turns to the east, and is raised slightly off the ground as you push your body to the east. **The release of energy** is channeled through the right rear leg, up the back, and into the arms ending at the tip of the staff. The lead or left leg is bent slightly at the knee, pointing to the east.

## Appellation #7

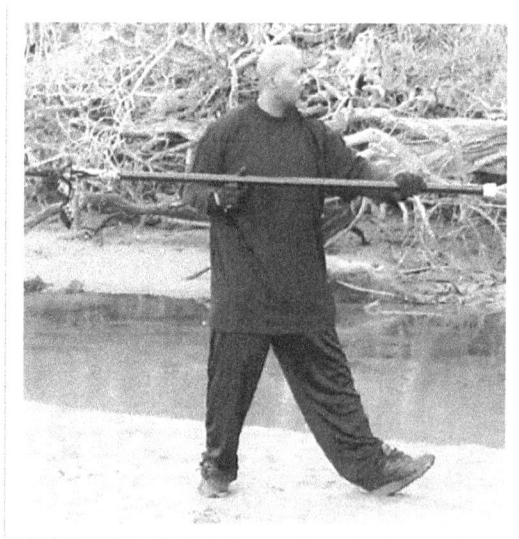

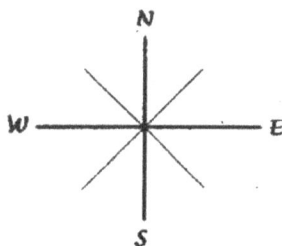

Right Ft.        Left Ft.

**#9 Diligent Crane rotates his beak -** While still facing east, the left hand releases the bottom of the staff. Twirl the staff counter clock-wise through the fingers of the right hand until the tip points west. Reengage and grab the bottom of the staff with the left hand.

### Appellation #8

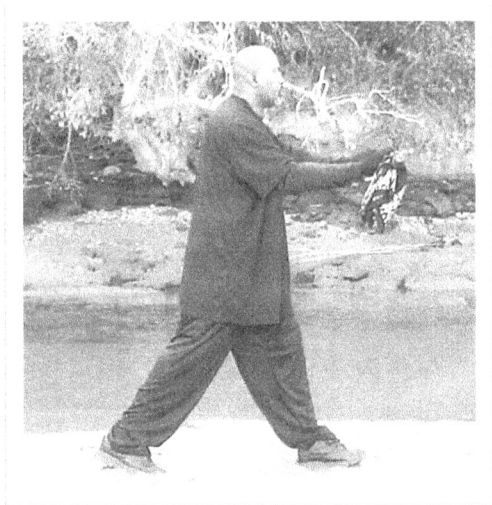

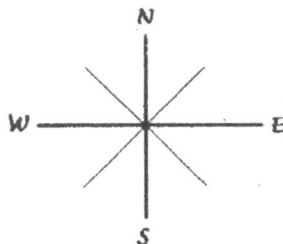

Right Ft.      Left Ft.

### Appellation #9

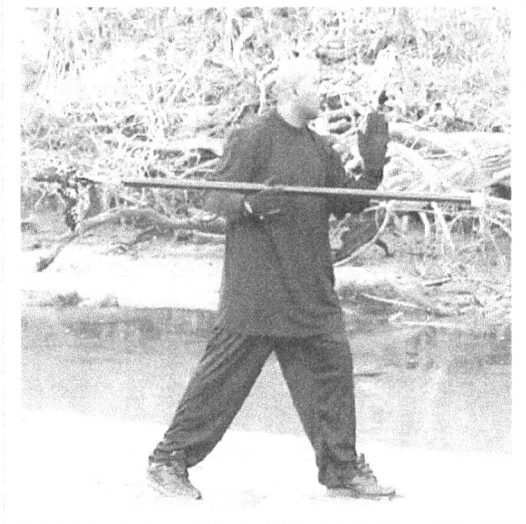

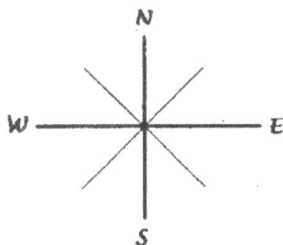

Right Ft.      Left Ft.

**#10 Divine bird looks to Heaven** - following the flow of energy the left foot raises off the ground and slides back behind the right leg as it touches the ground with the toes. (*The right foot is planted firmly to the ground*). Your body in response to this action bends over at the waist, still facing east. The movement ends as you drive the tip of the staff up into the air. The left hand holds the staff firmly at the bottom. The right hand is held firmly at the centre of the staff.

### Appellation #10

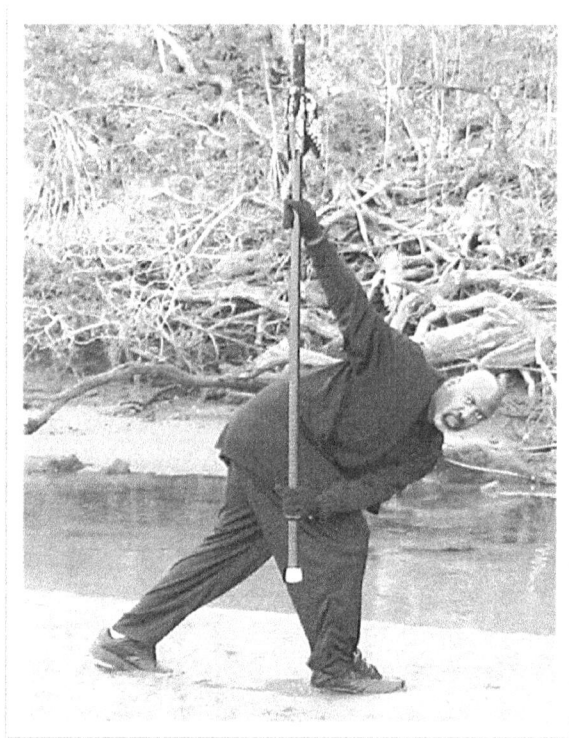

### Authors Note #1

When the left hand is holding the staff firmly at the bottom, your left arm is resting just above the right knee, and the right quadriceps. This is done to help secure the staff in position. The right hand acts as a balancing vector.

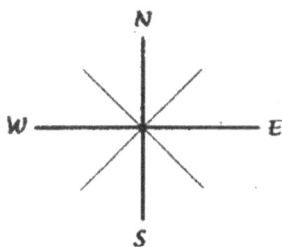

N
W — E
S

*Left Ft.*

*Right Ft.*

**#11 Ambitious Crane looks for food -** With inscrutable precision, you pull your entire body around in a counter clock-wise motion 180°. (*Distribute your weight between your left foot / instep, and the right foot / heel as you spin around to the left*). As the staff comes down the tip is pointing to the floor in **synchronicity** with the rotation of the body, following the flow of energy. The left hand is held at the base of the staff, while the right hand is positioned in the middle of the staff.

*Appellation #11*

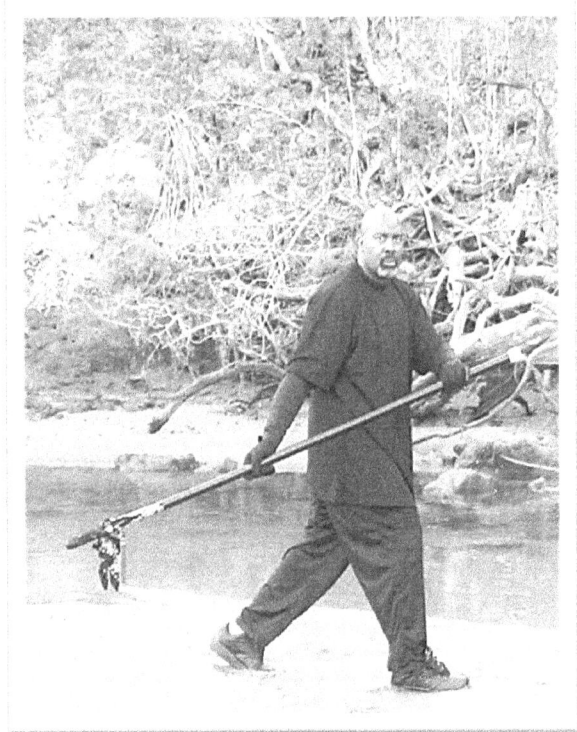

## Authors Note #2

When told to pull the body around, this is a spinning motion where both feet are in motion turning around to complete a 180° turn. This motion is carried throughout the body in sync, as your momentum is one complete action.

*Left Ft.*          *Right Ft.*

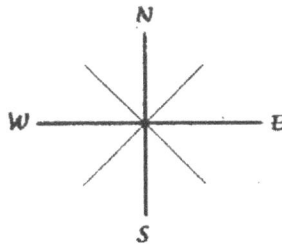

# Exercise Segment – Three

**#12 Heroic bird stretches his wings -** As the release of energy is followed, let the flow carry the staff around, as you stand upright. Facing west, with the staff behind your back, your arms should be held over your head; right hand under left griping the base of the staff. The tip of the staff should point down, at 45˚. (*The left foot leads the right foot in stagnation*).

## Appellation #12

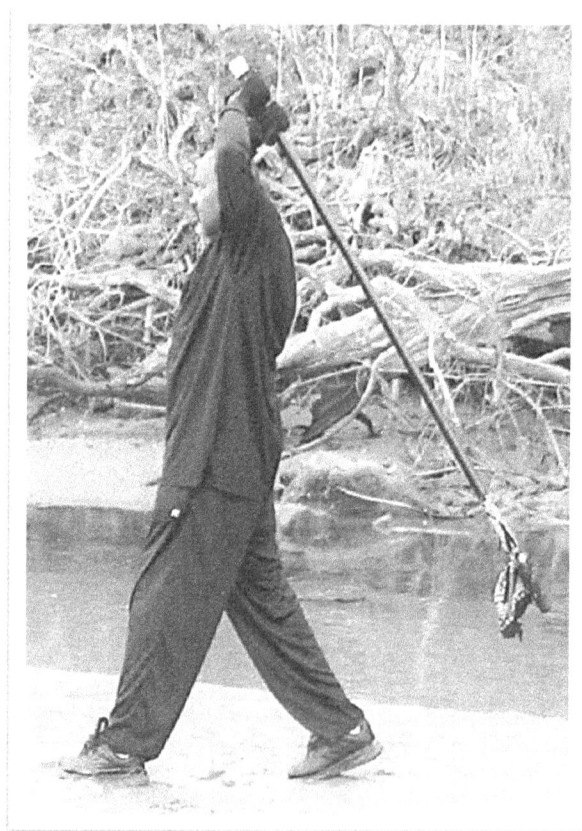

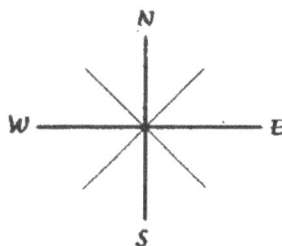

Left Ft.     Right Ft.

**#13 Uncanny Crane stomps his foot** - The left foot takes a step back about 40″ (*left foot pointing south*). In motion, the body drops down as far as possible. The right leg is held straight, with the toes pointing up. Bringing the staff overhead, you establish your balance on your left foot, as the left and right hand guide the staff to the floor in a semi-circle. (***Vertically***).

**#14 Fearless bird grabs a fish** - A jabbing motion, poking in & out.

*Right Ft.*     *Left Ft.*

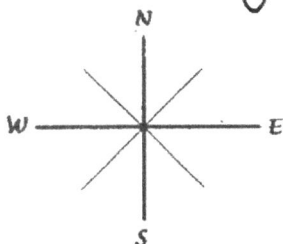

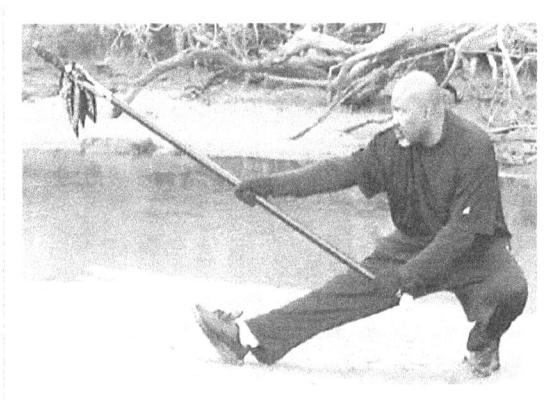

*Right Ft.*     *Left Ft.*

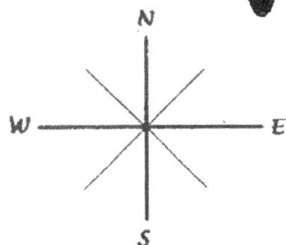

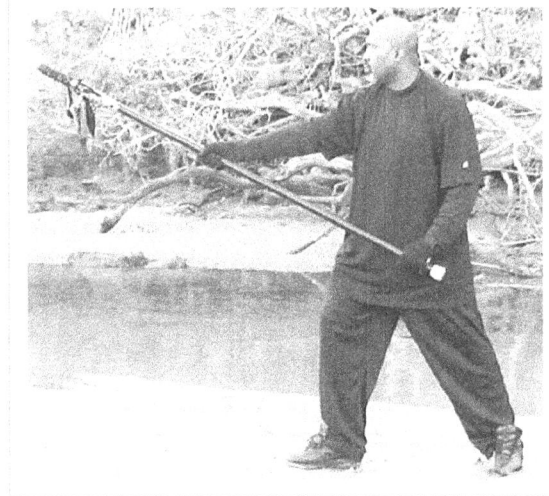

#15 A poignant bird embraces the new day - A. The right leg relaxes slightly, followed by the left hand reaching in at **proximal**. **B.** As you loosen your grip in the right hand, execute a figure eight in **proximal** of the body. Reach out with your left hand and finish the figure eight with the left hand, pulling the staff back behind the left side of the body. **C.** Raise your right hand above your head in **supination** and in harmony with the left leg, as it rises up to a 90° angle with the foot pointing downward. The staffs tip points down.

*Appellation #15 A.B.C.*

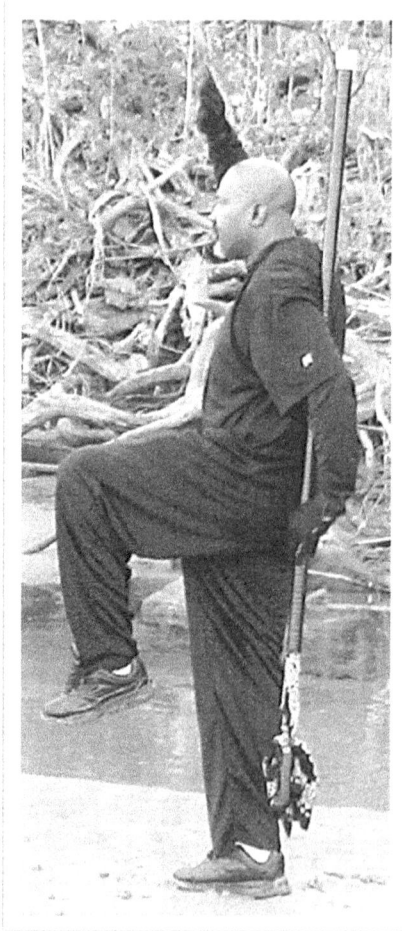

### Authors Note #3

As the left foot is raised, its energy is released from the previous position, carrying its energy into the next exercise. This is one fluid motion.

*Right Ft.* ⬭

*Left Ft.* ⬬

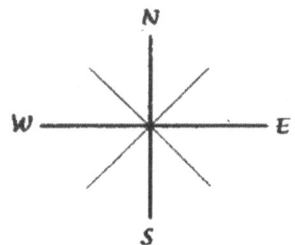

**#16 Insightful crane sweeps to the west** – Bring the right hand down in a clock-wise motion behind your back, and grab the staff out of your left hand with the right hand, and sweep the staff tip to the west. Your left leg is raised in a 90° angle, bent from the knee, with your left foot pointing down.

*Appellation #16*

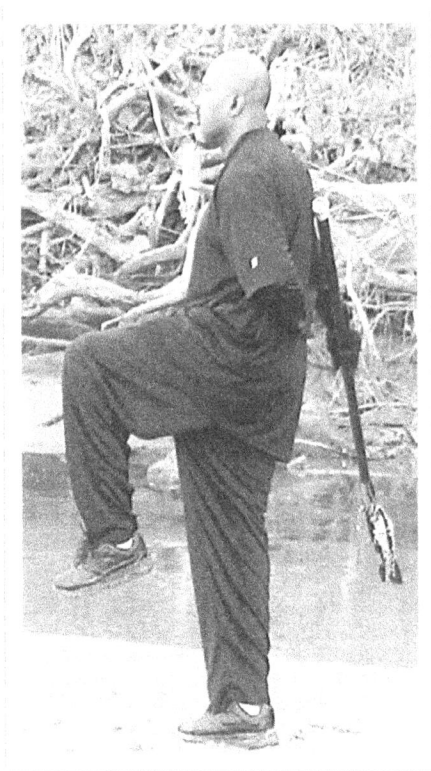

## Authors Note #4

Notice in exercises #1, #16, and #18, when told to go behind the back and grab the staff, this is a fluid motion. You release your grip in the left hand slightly, and allow the staff to slide down into the right hand. At which time you follow through and absorb the energy given, carrying it out and around to the next appellation. (*We equate energy to the Chinese term* **JING**).

*Right Ft.* ⬭

*Left Ft.* ⬬

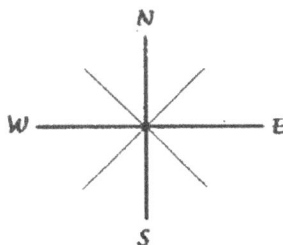

# Exercise Segment – Four

**#17A. <u>Lofty bird goes down under</u> -** Step forward with the left foot, and spin 180° about-face to the east. While in harmony, execute a figure eight with the staff, as you reach out with the left hand, and tuck the staff under your left arm, and shoulder (*the tip of the staff should be pointing to the north*). **#17B.** The right leg sweeps back past the left foot, (*toes to the floor*). Bending 90° @ the waist to the east, you bring the right hand out in **supination,** while pointing to the south. You should be looking to the north.

### Appellation #17A.                              #17B.

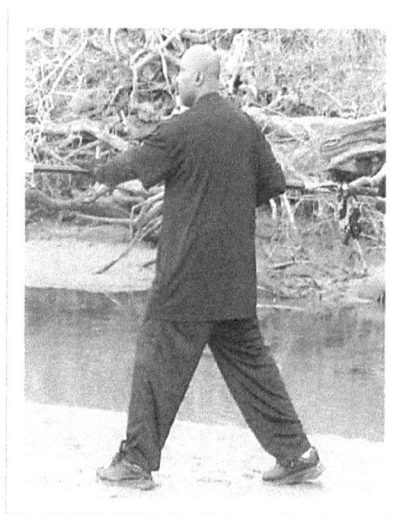

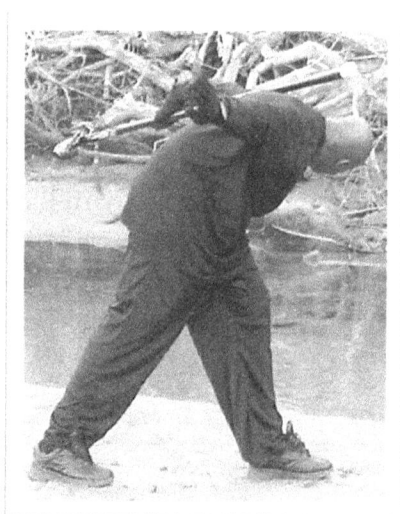

*Right Ft.*        *Left Ft.*

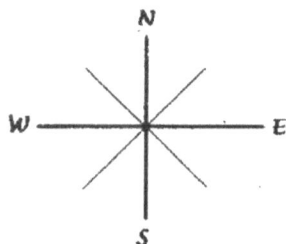

**#18A. Crane spreads his right wing open** - The right foot relaxes, and takes a step forward resting 12″ in front of the left leg. **#18B.** The right hand goes behind the back, and grabs the staff out of the left hand, sweeping across the south and raising the staff up above the head. (*The tip of the staff is pointing down -n- out*). While in harmony, your left leg is raised to a 90° angle as your body returns to the upright position-standing vertical with the right foot planted firmly on the floor.

*Appellation #18A.*            *#18B.*

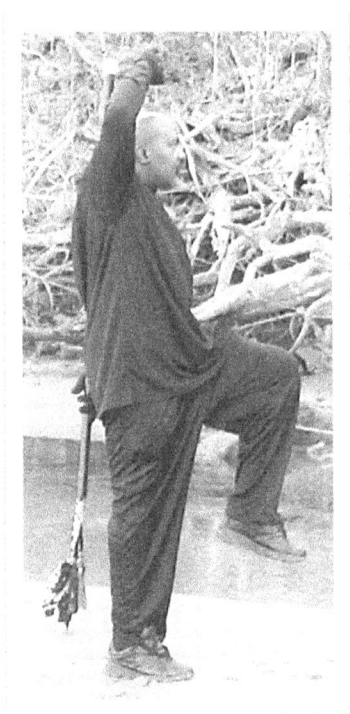 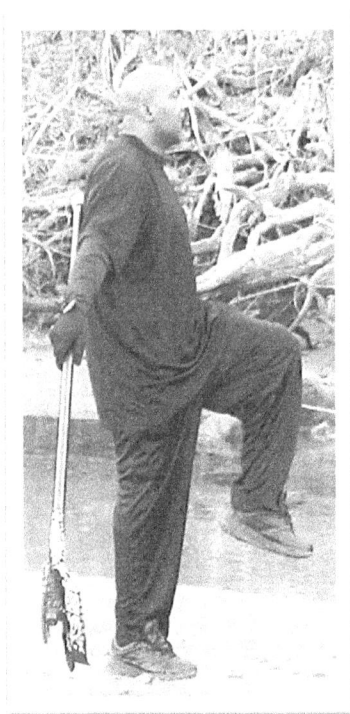

*Left Ft.* ⬤

*Right Ft.* ⬭

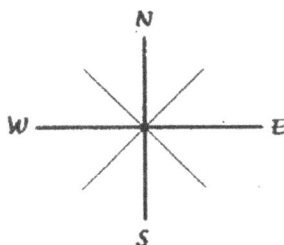

**#19 Angry bird flaps his wings -** Still standing vertically on the right foot, your left leg is bent at a 90° angle, with the knee bent and the foot pointing down. Your hands should be up above your head twirling the staff, until it comes to rest on the left shoulder just behind your neck.

Left Ft.

Right Ft.

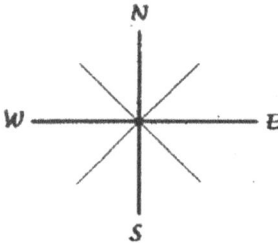

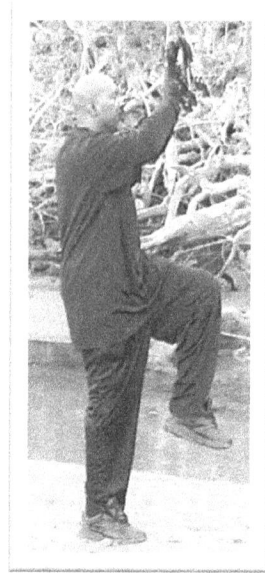

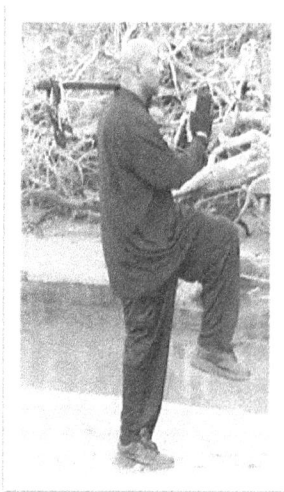

Left Ft.

Right Ft.

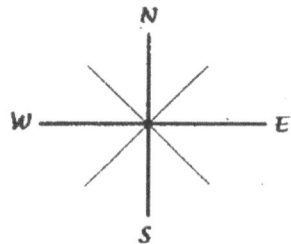

# #20 The agile bird points to the south.

Pausing only for a second. The staff should now be resting on your left shoulder with the left hand about, 12″ – 16″ from the bottom of the staff as it points south. Your left leg is still bent 90° at the knee, with the right foot firmly on the ground. The right hand is placed in the center of the chest at **proximal**. **Alt. move**. (*Take the staff and twirl it 360° around the neck with the left hand catching it on the left side with your right hand*). Follow the flow of energy. Carry the staff back to the right side of the body. Once again resuming at, **The Ready Position**.

## The Ready Position
*Alpha & Omega*

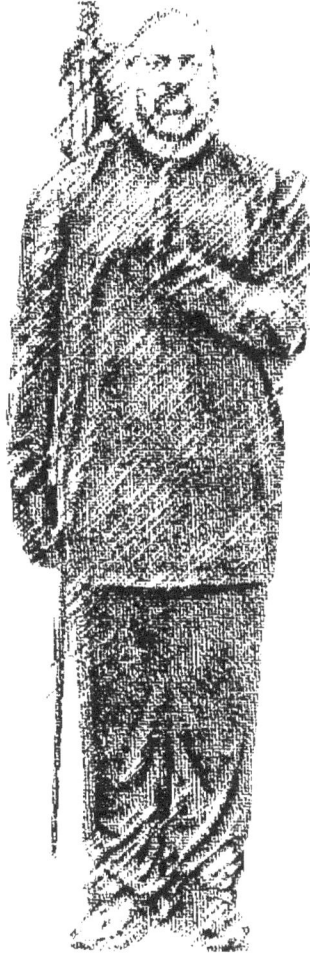

## Authors Note #5

*The completion of the exercise ends with you facing to the east. At this point, you can continue to repeat the entire routine again, or stop.* **If you decide to stop, reposition yourself back at,** *The Ready Position* **facing south.**

## *Alpha & Omega*
## THE READY POSITION

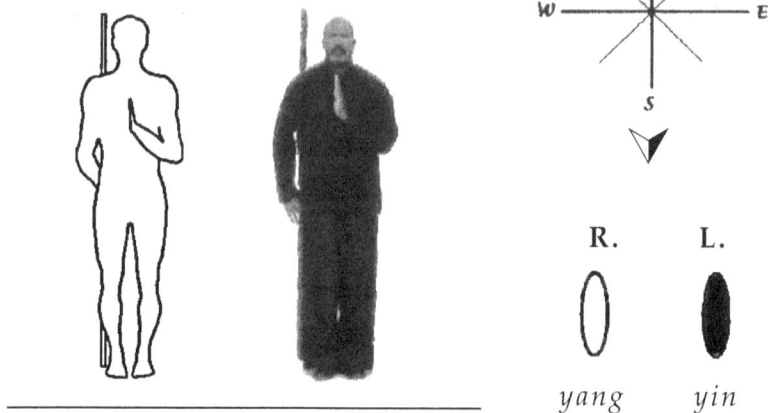

R.  L.

yang  yin

Starting in **The Ready Position**, follow the numbers above each form as it carries you through the exercise segments, step by step.

3.

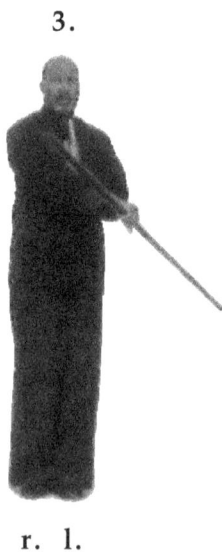

r.  l.

4.

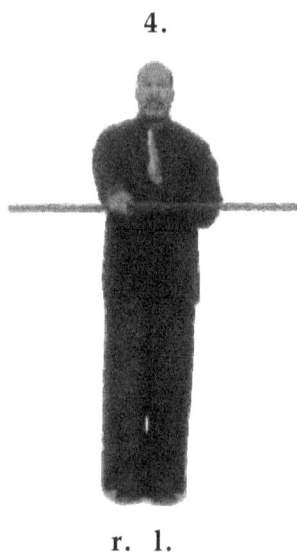

r.  l.

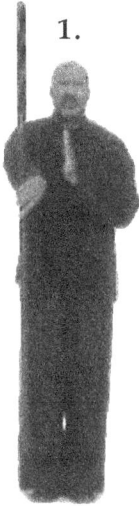

1.

r.  l.

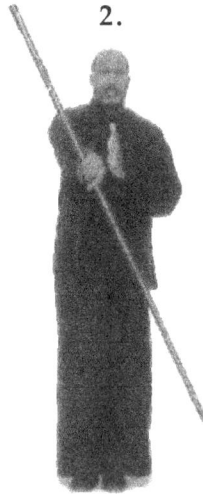

2.

r.  l.

**#1-#11**Execute a figure-8 twirling the staff in front of your body. As previously mentioned, this is a controlled release of energy.

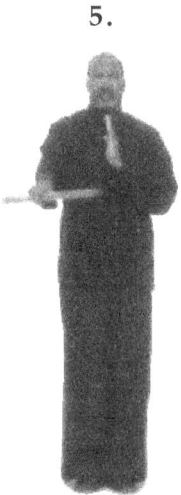

5.

r.  l.

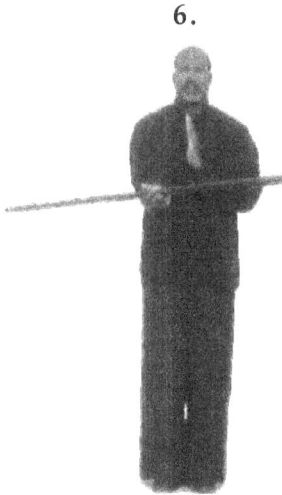

6.

r.  l.

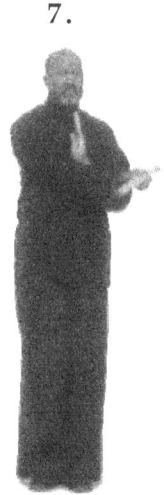

7.

r.  l.

**8.**

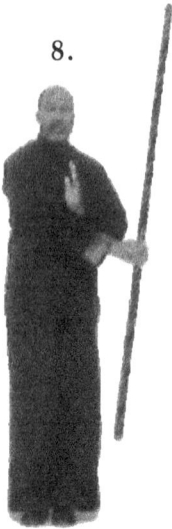

r.  l.

**9.**

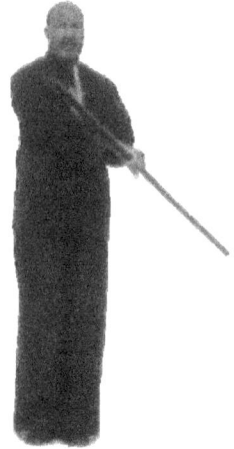

r.  l.

**#12** The right leg rises as you Salute the Heavens, then lowers.

#12 **Salute The Heavens.**

**12.**

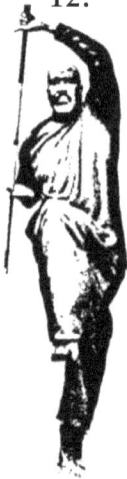

r.  l.

**13.**

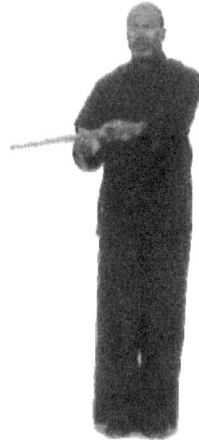

r.  l.

**Figure-8** *(#1-#11)*

**10.**

r.  l.

**11.**

r.  l.

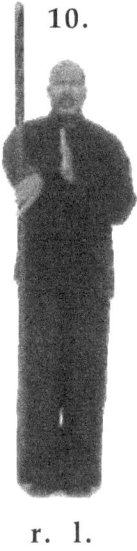

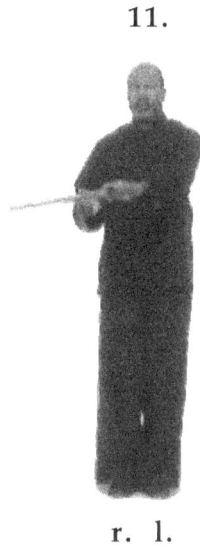

**#13-#23** Execute a figure-8 twirling the staff in front of your body.

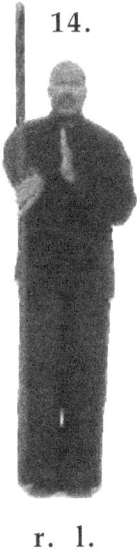

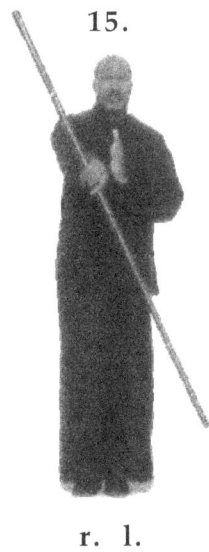

**14.**

r.  l.

**15.**

r.  l.

16.

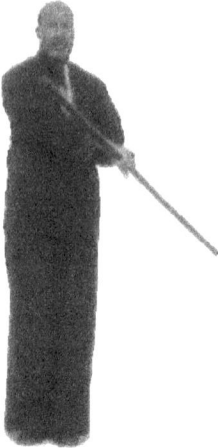

r. l.

17.

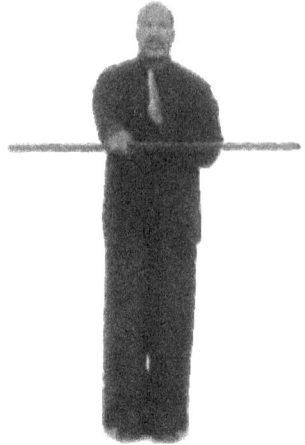

r. l.

**#13-#23** Execute a figure eight with the staff in front of your body. Let the energy of the staff flow freely, and easily around.

20.

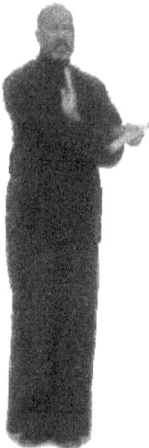

r. l.

21.

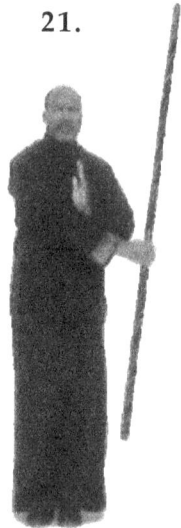

r. l.

**Figure-8** *(#13-#23)*

18.

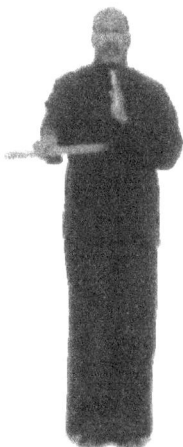

r.  l.

19.

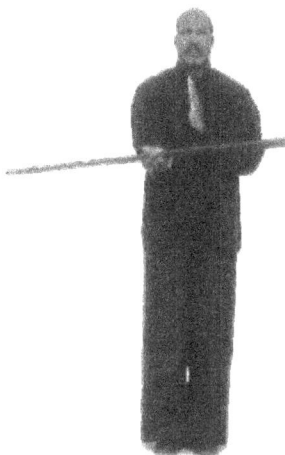

r.  l.

**#23** Begin to tuck the staff under your left shoulder, as you bring the left foot up in sync along with the right hand.

22.

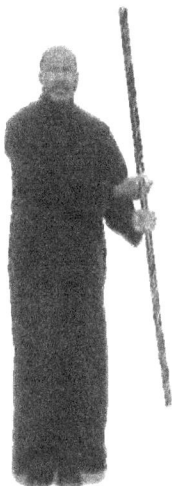

r.  l.

23.

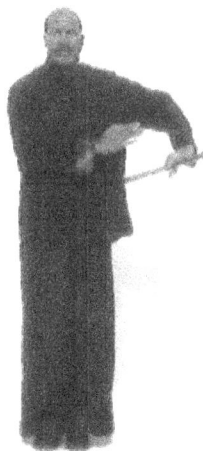

r.  l.

## #24 Embrace The New Day.    #25 Secure the right wing.

24.                              25.

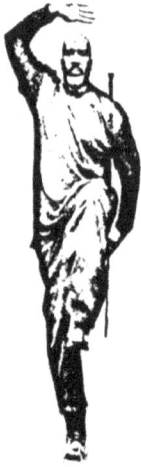        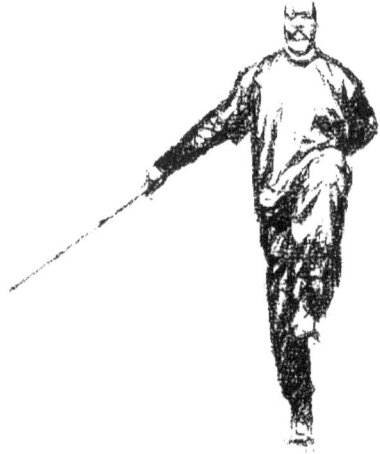

r.  l.                           r.  l.

## #28 Powerful bird holds up the sky.

28.

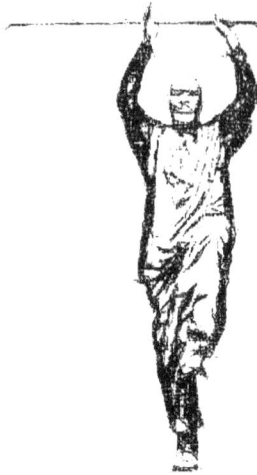

r.  l.

**26.**

**27.**

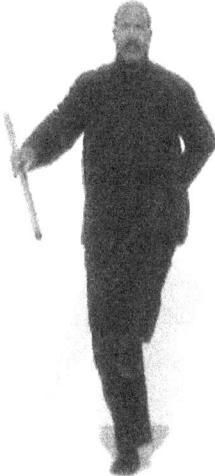

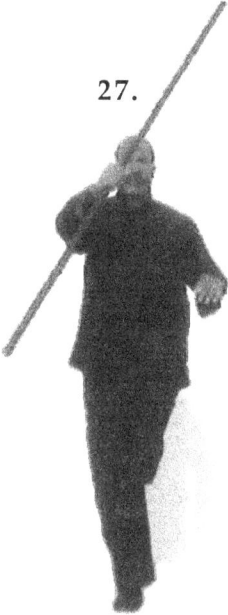

r.  l.

r.  l.

**#29** From the south position, you rotate 90° degrees to the east from the waist. As the left leg lowers, you touch heel to toe, with the left foot pointing east. The right foot points to the south.

**29.**

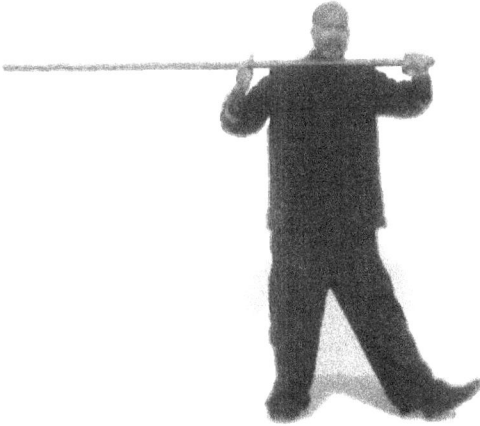

r.          l.

# EXERCISE SEGMENT 2. Facing East (#30-#41)

#30 **Advance to release.**    #31 **Immaculate bird strikes his prey.**

### 30.

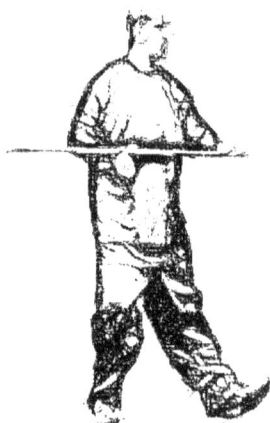

r.        l.

### 31.

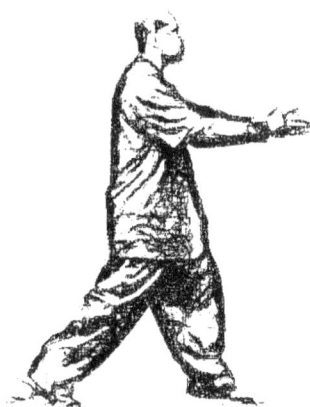

r.        l.

**#31** The heel of the right foot turns to the east, and rises slightly off the ground as you push your body to the east. Also known as, Releasing.

### 34.

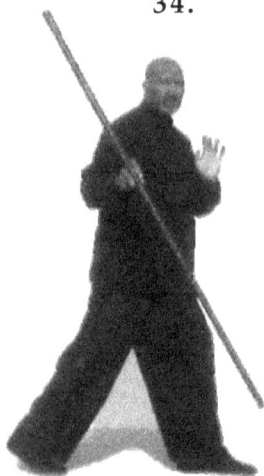

r.        l.

### 35.

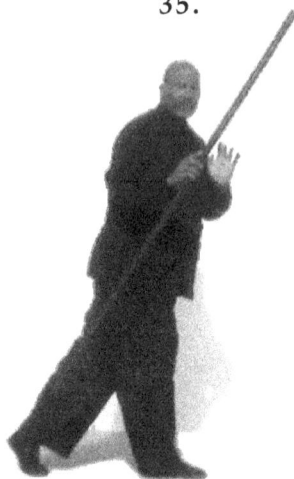

l.        r.

## #32 Diligent Crane rotates his beak.

32.

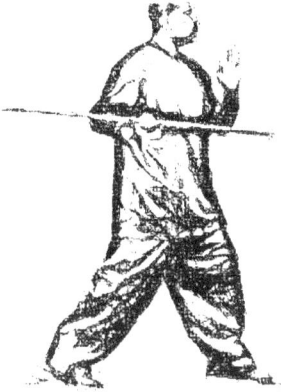

33.

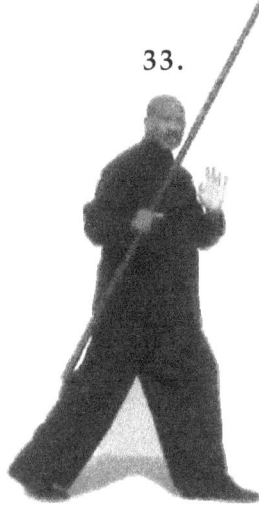

r.        l.              r.        l.

#36 Following the flow of energy the left foot rises off the ground, and slides back behind the right leg as it touches the ground with the toes.

## #37 Divine bird looks to Heaven.

36.

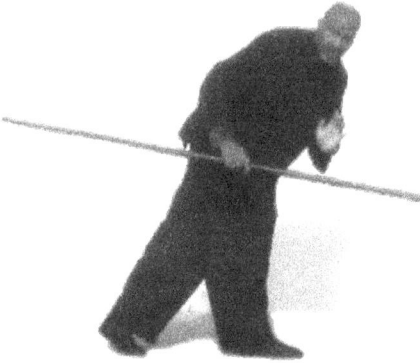

37.

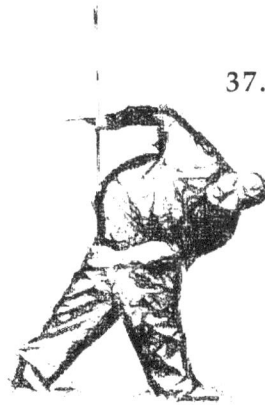

l.        r.              l.        r.

**Facing East** *(#30-#41)*

38.   39.

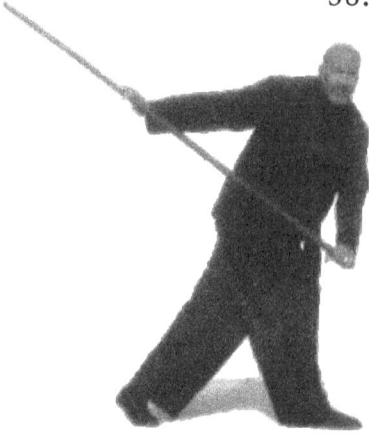
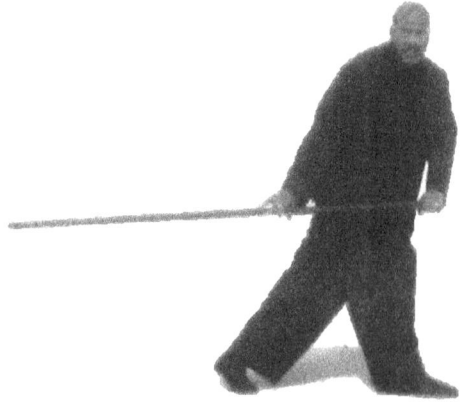

l.   r.   l.   r.

#38-#45 You pull your entire body around in a counter clock-wise motion 180° to the right. As the staff comes down, the tip points to the floor. The rotation of your body follows the flow of energy.

**Facing West** *(#42-#45)*

42.   43.

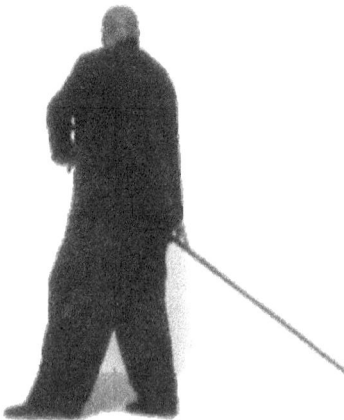
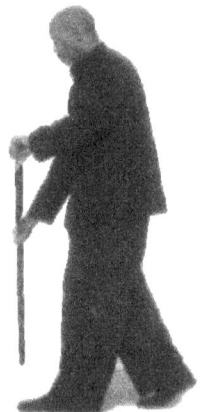

l.   r.   l.   r.

#40 Ambitious Crane looks for food.

40.     41.

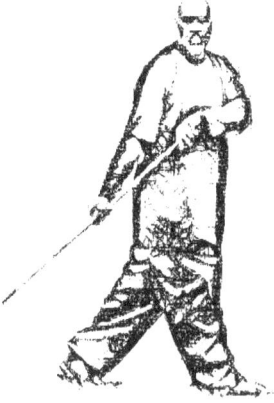 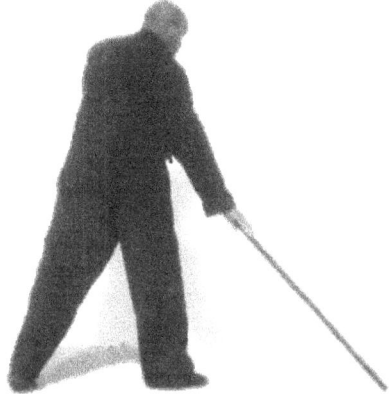

l.  r.  l.  r.

When told to pull the body around, this is a spinning motion where both feet are in motion turning around to complete a 180° turn. This motion is carried throughout the body in sync.

44.     45.

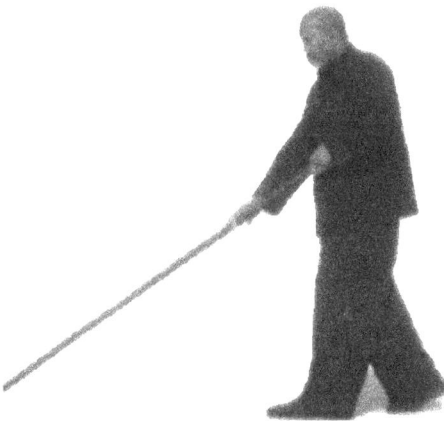 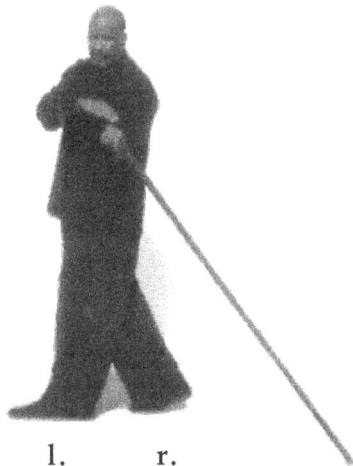

l.  r.  l.  r.

## # 46 Heroic bird stretches his wings.

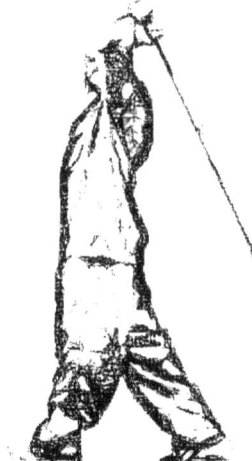

46.

l.      r.

**#46** Facing west, with the staff behind your back, your arms should be held over your head; right hand under left griping the base of the staff.

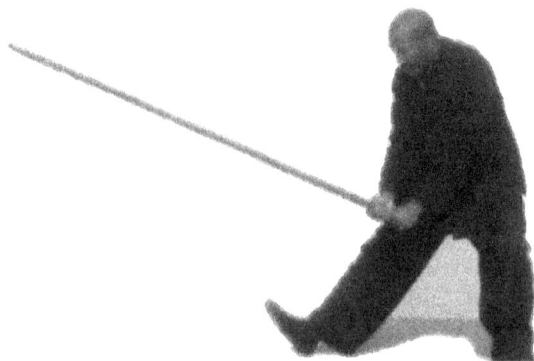

48.

r.      l.

## Overhead Strike *(#46-#49)*

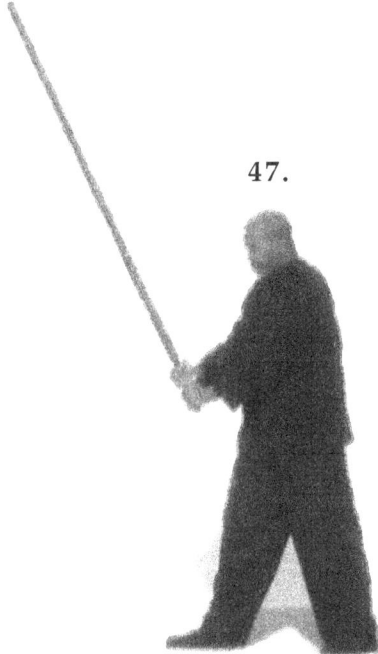

47.

r.              l.

#49 The left foot takes a step back about 40" (_left foot pointing south_). The right leg is held straight, with the toes pointing up. Bringing the staff overhead, you establish balance on your left foot.

### # 49 Uncanny Crane stomps his foot.

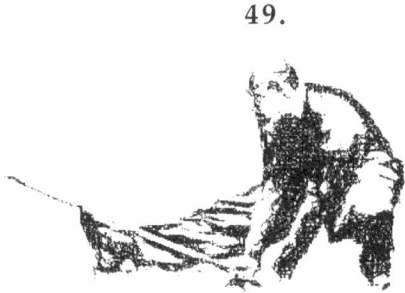

49.

r.                    l.

**50.**

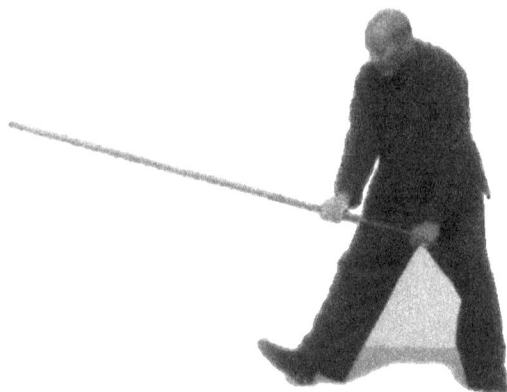

r.                    l.

**#50-#53** As you bring the staff back up to a ready position, with the left hand begin an ambidextrous jabbing movement.

**52.**

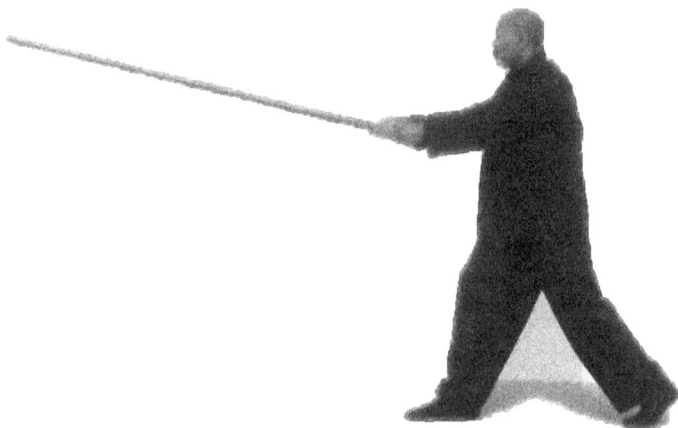

r.                    l.

# 51 Fearless bird grabs a fish.

51.

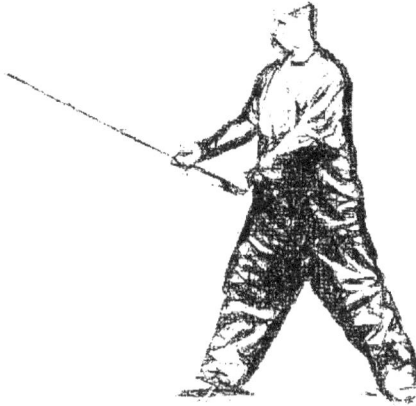

r                    l.

Switching from left to right, repeat the jab until you are
satisfied. Upon completion, you return to a ready position. #53

53.

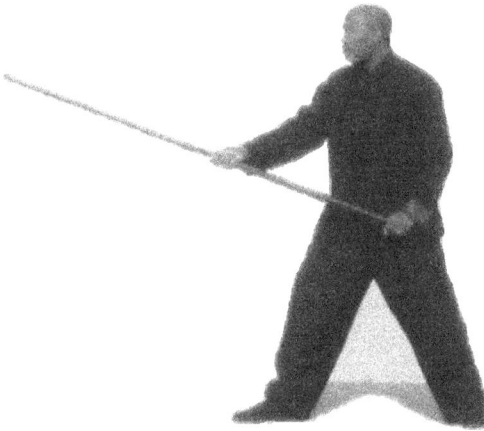

r.                    l.

54.

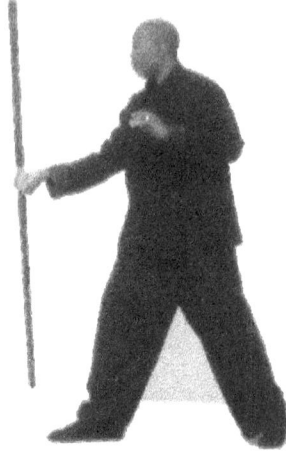

r.                    l.

**#54-#63** Execute a figure eight with the staff in the right had. As you reach out with the left hand, tuck the staff under your left arm, and shoulder.

56.

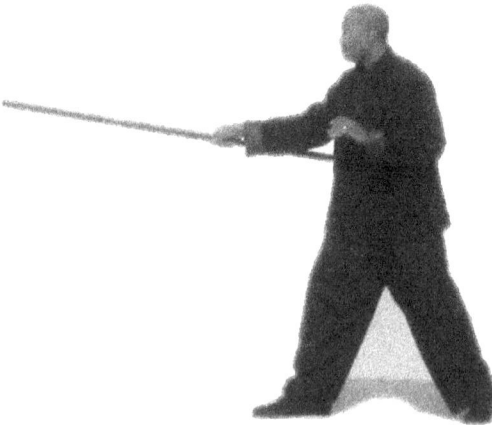

r.                    l.

**Figure-8** *(#54-#63)*

**55.**

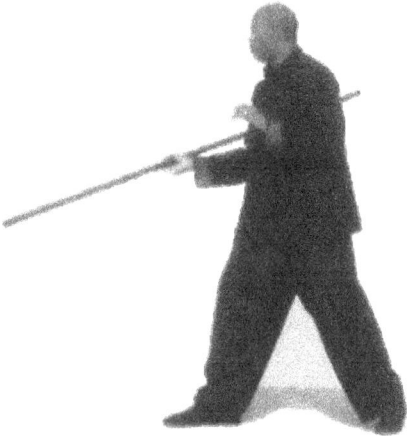

r.        l.

**#54-#63** This is a continuous flow of energy. There is little to no movement at all from the left hand, until it reaches out.

**57.**

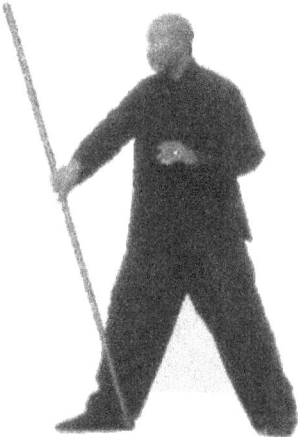

r.        l.

58.

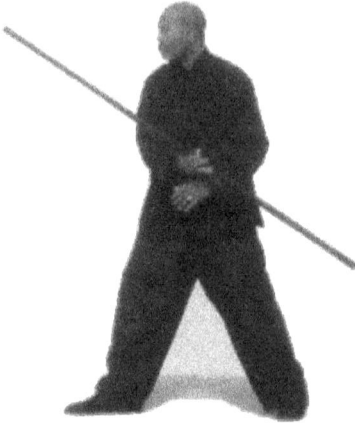

r.　　　　l.

59.

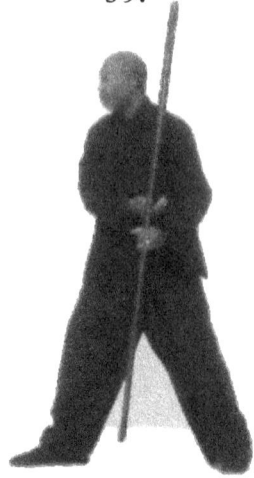

r.　　　　l.

**#58-#60** Follow the energy of the staff as it comes around.

**# 63 A poignant bird embraces the new day.**

62.

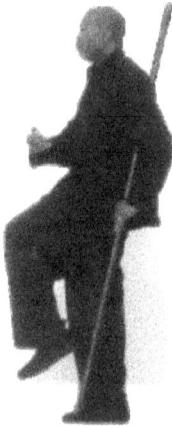

l.　r.

63.

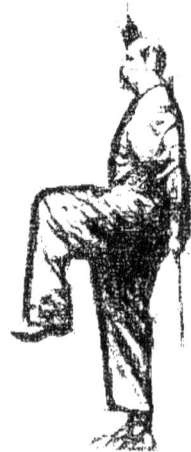

l.　　r.

**Figure-8** *(#54-#63)*

60.

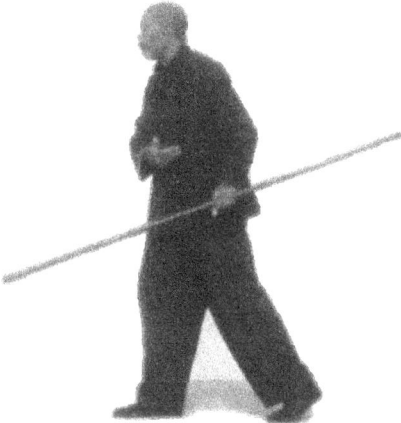

r.          l.

61.

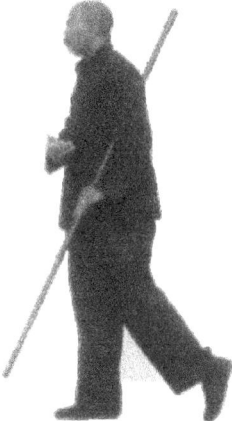

r.          l.

#60-#63 Absorb the energy, and carry it through the body.

# 64 Insightful Crane sweeps to the west.

64.

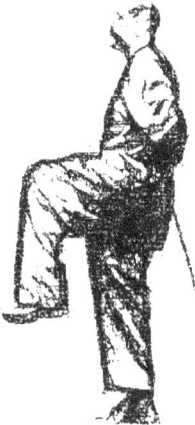

l.          r.

65.

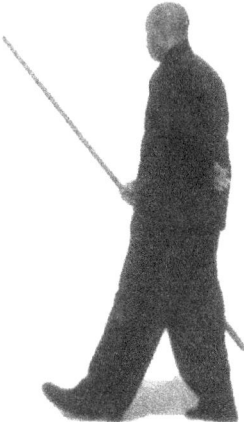

l.          r.

## EXERCISE SEGMENT 4. Facing East (#66-#87)

#67 Lofty bird goes down under. A.

66.

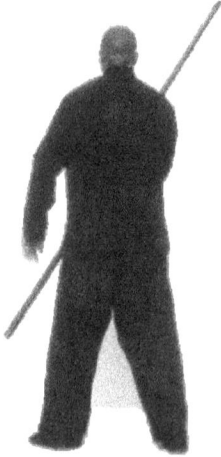

l.       r.

67.

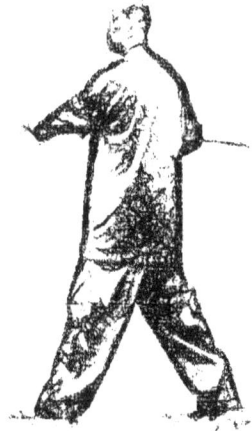

l.       r.

#64-#69 As the staff wraps around your body, let the energy turn you around until you are facing to the east, bending over slightly.

70.

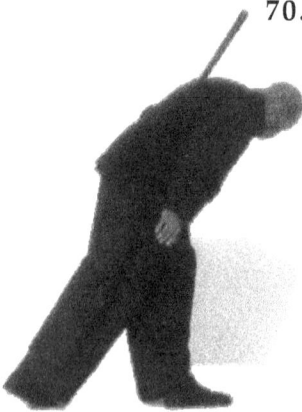

r.       l.

#71 Lofty bird goes down under. B.

71.

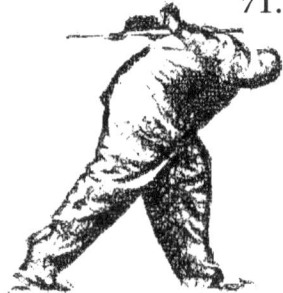

r.       l.

68.                                    69.

l.          r.              r.          l.

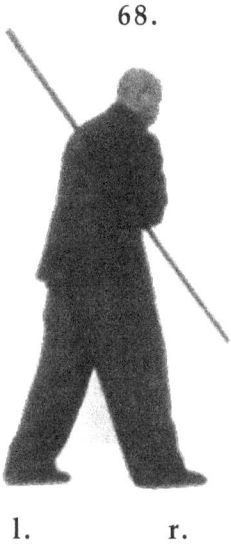

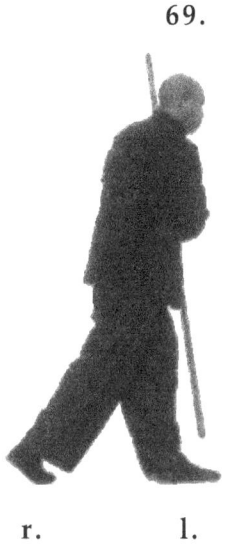

#**69-#71** Slide the right foot behind the left foot, with the toes touching the floor. Bend 90° degrees at the waist, and release your energy throughout your body evenly. #**73** Step forward with the right foot.

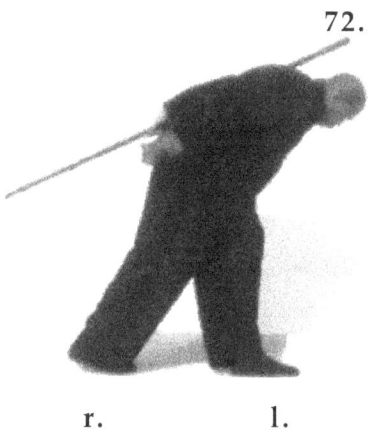

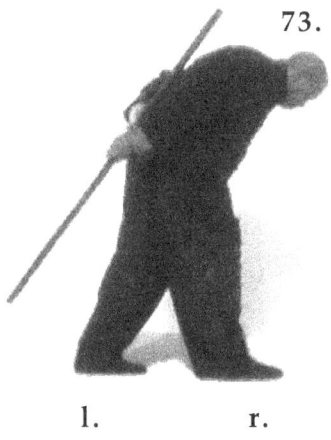

72.                                    73.

r.          l.              l.          r.

# #74 Crane spreads his right wing open.  A. & B.

### 74.

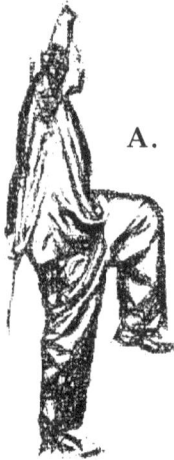

A.

r.        l.

### 75.

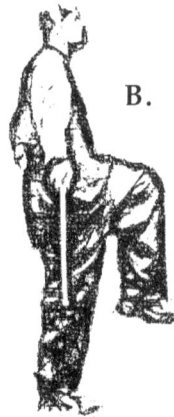

B.

r.        l.

# #78 Angry bird flaps his wings.

### 78.

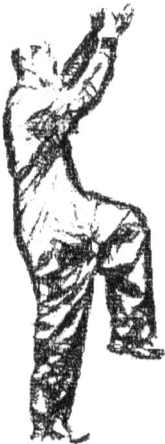

r.        l.

### 79.

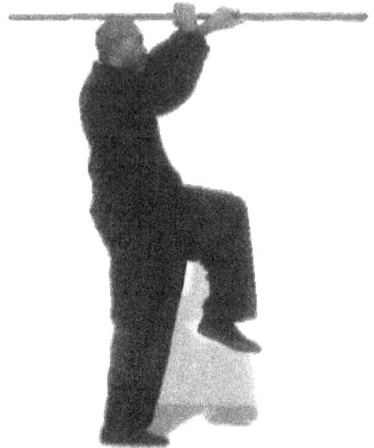

r.        l.

**Facing East** *(#66-#87)*

**76.**

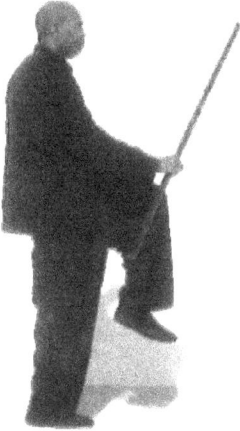

r.    l.

**77.**

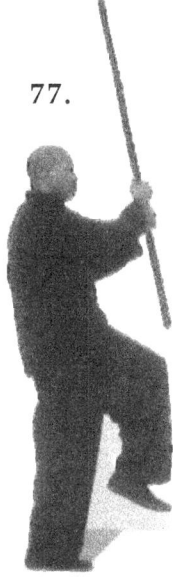

r.    l.

**#74-#80** Following the flow of energy, the staff is carried around the body to the right side, and twirled above the head.

**80.**

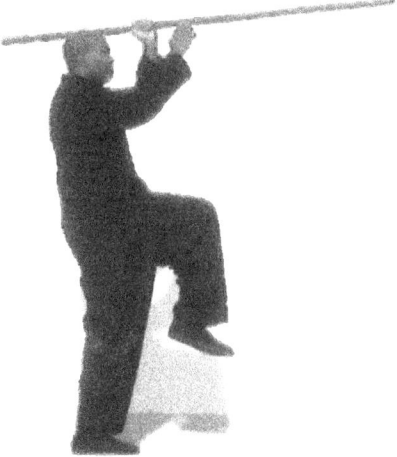

r.    l.

**81.**

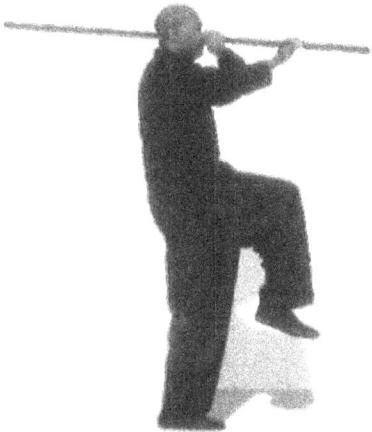

r.    l.

## #82 The agile bird points to the south.

82.

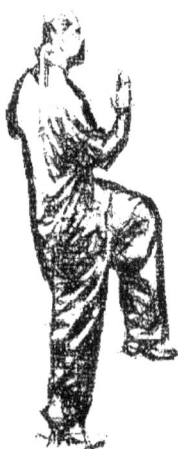

r.    l.

83.

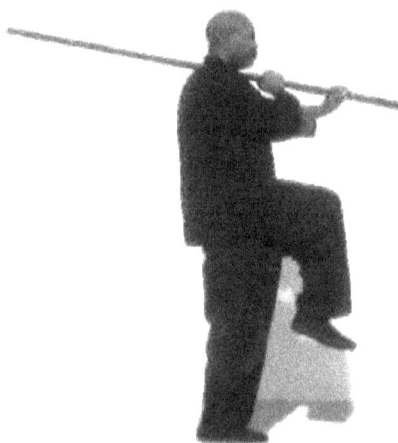

r.    l.

#82-#87 The final release of energy begins as you remove the staff from behind your neck, tucking it under your right shoulder.

86.

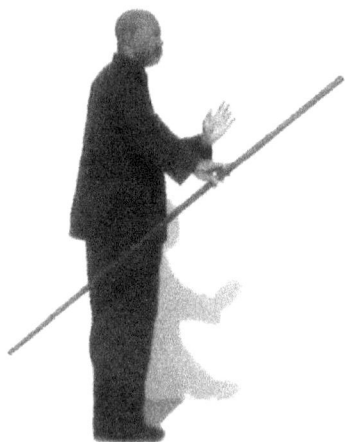

r. & l.

87.

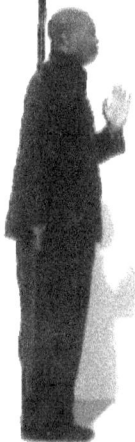

r. & l.

88.

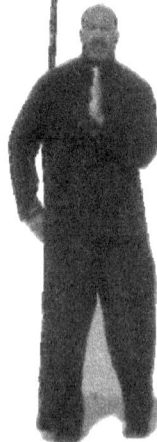

r.    l.

84.

85.

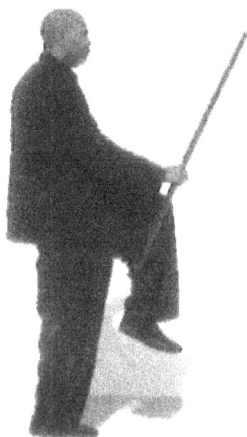

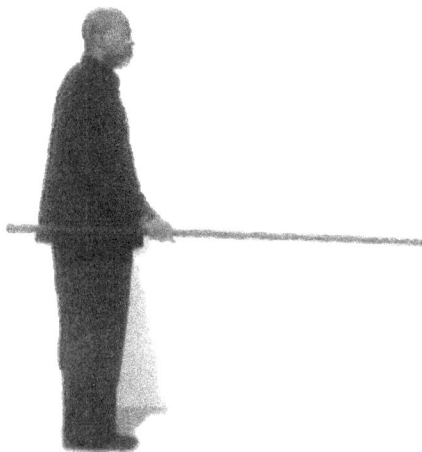

r.     l.

r. & l.

As you near the end of the exercise as in previous examples, you have the option to start over, or end the exercise facing east #87.

*Alpha & Omega*
**THE READY POSITION**

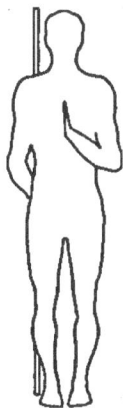

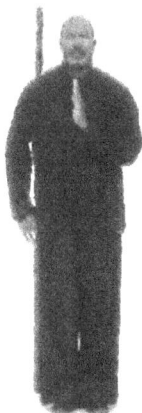

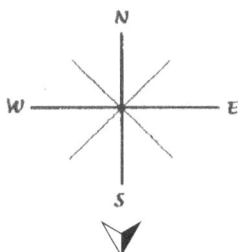

R.       L.

yang     yin

# Chapter #3 Review

**The Spear** (Qiang) - *The King of Long Weapons*

**The Staff** (Gun) - *The Father of all Weapons*

**Spear & Staff** - Qiang & Gun *(Chinese; pinyin)* = SPEAR & STAFF

**Variations**

---

**The Basic Stance**

*F = ma*

**The Five Elements**

**The Four Corners**

**The Shuffle**

**The Side Step**

*Definition #1*

*Definition #2*

**Intangible Motion**

**Exercise Segment – One**
**Exercise Segment – Two**
**Exercise Segment – Three**
**Exercise Segment – Four**

# THE CRANE

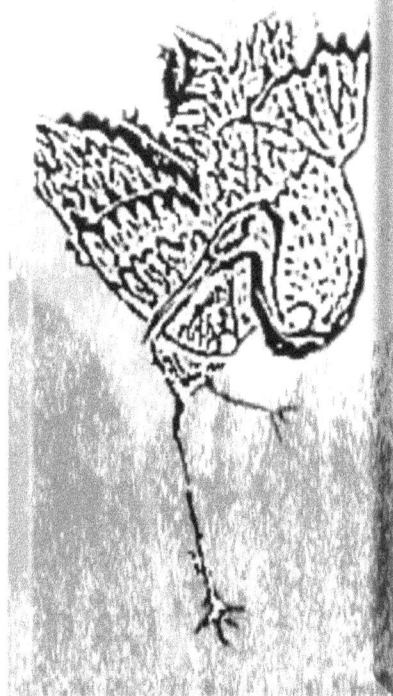

方法是本能的无意识的。

方法就是与众不同的意识。

通常会丢失，而渴望找到

**The Way is often lost, but aspires to be found.**

The Way is distinctively *conscious.*
The Way is instinctively *unconscious.*

# Chapter

# 4.

## The Walking Stick & Cane
ROM - *or* - *a.k.a.* (ROME)

## The Crane Form *Part 3*
## Simplified Daily Exercise Routine

---

When the spirit is disturbed,
its flow is given a haven.

To neutralize the act,
you must surmise an intervention.

Release,
the abode....

# Walking Stick & Cane

"Cane" _stems from biblical Hebrew_ - (Qana)

_The difference in sticks, and canes is in the material used. Sticks were traditionally made of ivory, whalebone, ebony, and other precious items, whereas canes were made from malacca, rattan, bamboo, and other resilient reeds._ **(This list also included certain metals, steel, aluminum, and brass).**

**The Walking Stick and The Common Cane,** is the most readily available implement in your arsenal. It can change from a simple walking apparatus, to a deadly weapon of choice within seconds. Because of this, it is quite often considered an infamous, and praised tool.

Within the dominions of combat, it is often used in close quarter settings to subdue an opponent, or it can be whirled around in a whipping like manner, much like the staff.

**The Cane**
**Metal -** (_3ft. 36in._)

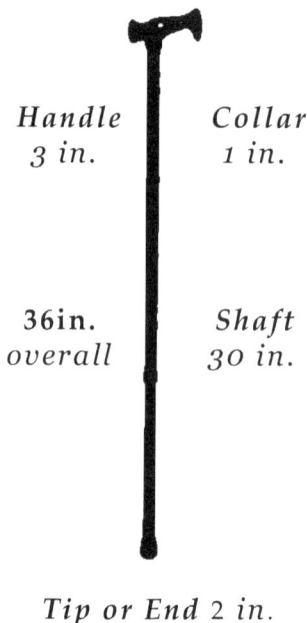

_Handle_
_3 in._

_Collar_
_1 in._

**36in.**
_overall_

_Shaft_
_30 in._

_Tip or End_ 2 in.

The cane is invaluable as it can break _bones, finger joints, knuckles, and bony portions of the upper hand. Other areas include the wrist, elbow, collarbone, and jawbone, along with the bridge of the nose, and temple._ Such blows, or strikes can detain, disable, or cause death.

## The Walking Stick
*Bamboo* - (*4ft. 48in.*)

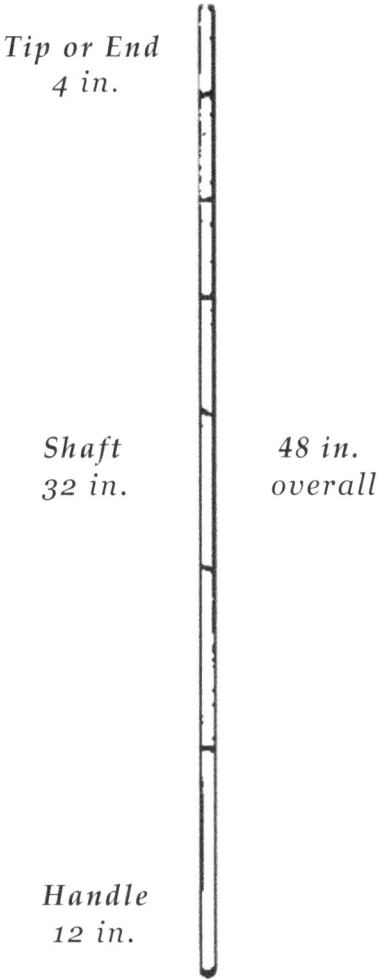

*Tip or End*
*4 in.*

*Shaft*
*32 in.*

*48 in.*
*overall*

*Handle*
*12 in.*

In this our forth chapter, we will cover the practical applications of, **The Walking Stick and Cane,** as a wellness aid. In the confines of training, the first priority is to learn how to turn it into an extension of the mind, and body. The second focus is to understand how the stick is used, with conditioned reflexes of a natural response. Third is the adaptation of the natural order, which is the flow of energy. This is not a forced energy, but more of a calm relaxed; and unconscious flowing, of motion, and energy.

"Walking Stick" *stems from ancient Japan* - (Jo)

*Remember to take great caution and care, when applying the following techniques. The Walking Stick, and Cane like the Spear, and Staff are still formidable weapons, and should be given the proper respect that they are due.*

# Range of Motion

ROM - or - a.k.a. (ROME)

Range of motion exercises are also called **ROM** or what I like to call **ROME**. ROME's help to keep your muscles and joints healthy. These exercises consist of three types. **Active ROME's (***like the ones demonstrated in chapters 2, and 3***)** are done by a person without any help, whereas **Active-Assisted ROME's** are done by a person with the aid of a helper. **Passive ROME's** are done for a person by the helper. The helper does the ROME's because the person cannot do them under their own power. Do not attempt to do any of the exercises shown here; or any kind of fitness routine such as **Tai Chi** or **Chi Gong** without first talking to your doctor, or physical therapist. The two of you should be able to decide what exercise plan or fitness régimes are best. (*Keep in mind that the routines displayed in chapters two, and three, are **Active ROM's,** and apply to advanced students only*).

**ROM** or **ROME** is very important if you have been stricken ill, injured; or confined to a bed, and wheelchair. ROME's help keep the joints, tendons, ligaments, and muscles flexible, and lubricated. They also help to keep your joints supple. The execution of daily ROME's is a good way to keep blood flowing to the joint areas. This can also help prevent blood clots, which accumulate in the blood stream.

In order for the body to stay fit, a reasonable amount of exercise is needed. You will begin to notice your heart is stronger, and your breathing is more controlled. As the heart and lungs get stronger, blood flows more freely to the muscles, bones, and skin. The Increase of blood flow will send oxygen and nutrients to body tissues, and organs with ease.

A key factor to remember is to understand the range of motion of your body, and how it relates to the normal ranges of motion. This is done to avoid the threat of hyperextending a joint. Understanding the difference between outward rotation, (*external*) and inward rotation, (*internal*) will help you to avoid any further injury.

## THE ROM TEST *pgs.(153 - 161)*

**#1** *Start out by determining the range of motion in your arms. Lift your arms up slowly, from the sides until they reach above your head. Pay attention to any difficulty.* **When you feel pain, stop!**

**#2** *Raise your arms in front of you slowly, until they are extended above your head. Pay attention to any difficulty. If you are able to, proceed to #3.* **When you feel pain, stop!**

**#3** *Rotate each arm slowly in a clockwise motion. If for some reason you cannot complete a full circle, skip this evaluation and move on to #4. Once again, there is no need for you to cause any more pain or injury to yourself.* **When you feel pain, stop!**

**#4** *Lift each leg slowly from a seated position in front of you. As in the previous exercises, pay close attention to any difficulty in movement.* **When you feel pain, stop!**

**#5** *While sitting, rotate your head, and upper body to the left, and right slowly. Any motion that causes pain should be noted. This type of evaluation should be applied to other areas of the body as well. After words, you should consult your primary care doctor or physician. He may recommend Physical Therapy, a Specialist, or medicine to help with your limited range of motion. Either way it is important that you seek help as soon as possible.* **When you feel pain, stop!**

# RANGE OF MOTION

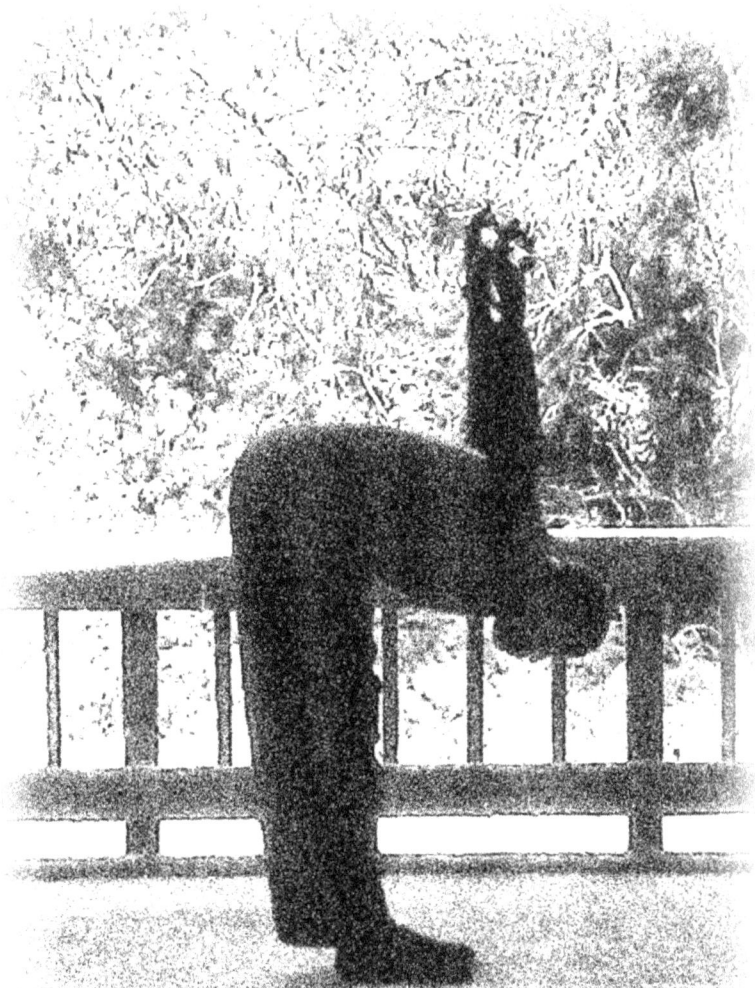

The Forward Hung

# #1 Lift arms slowly from the side.

#1

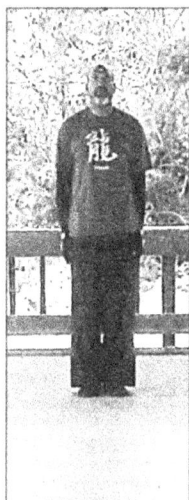

#2

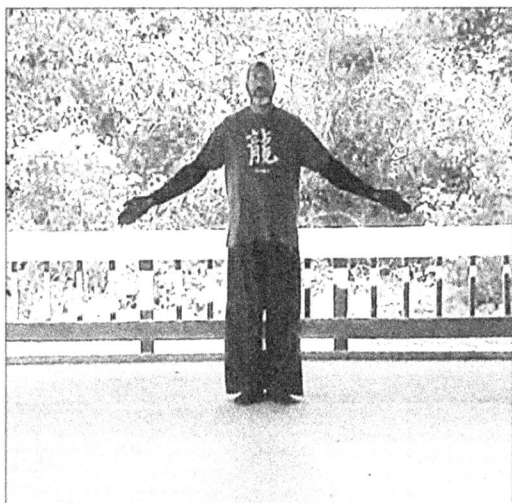

#3

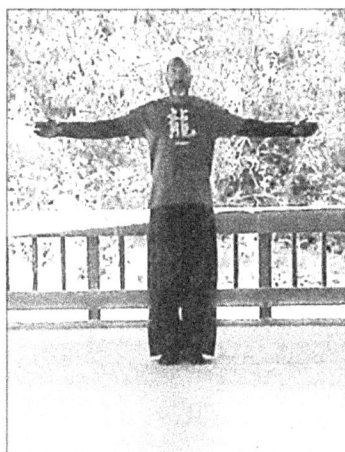

#4

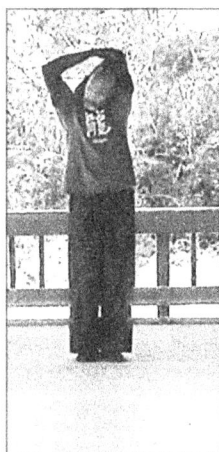

#5

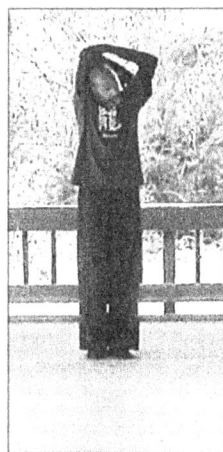

# #2 Lift arms in front of your body.

#1

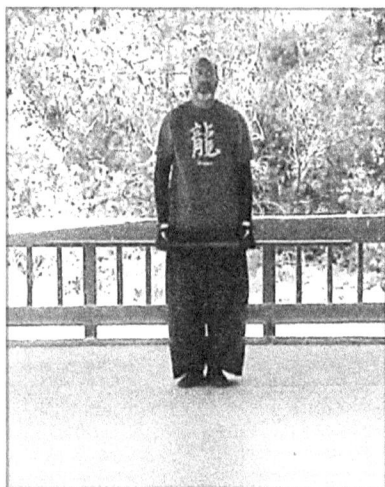

#2

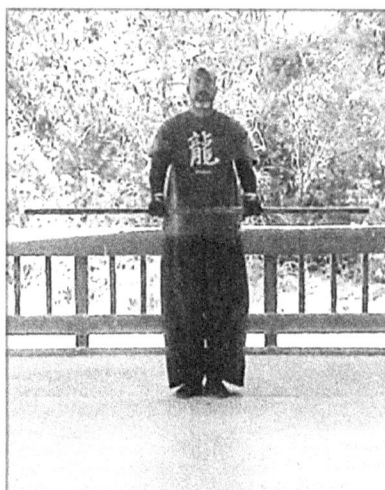

#3

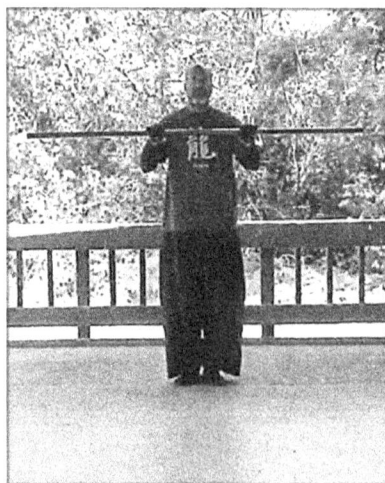

#4

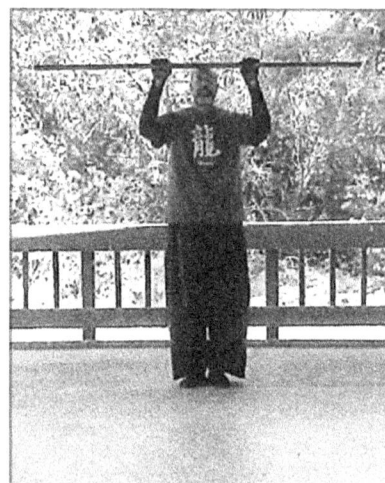

# #3 Rotate arms in a clockwise motion.

### #1

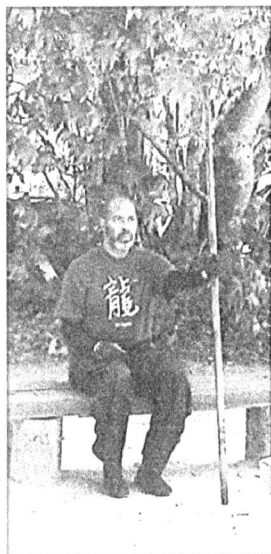

### #2

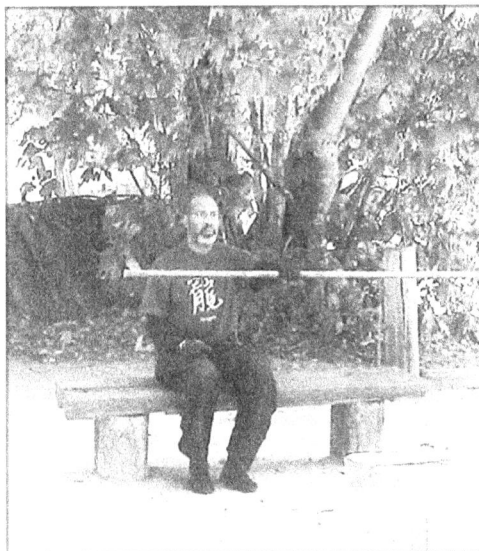

### #3

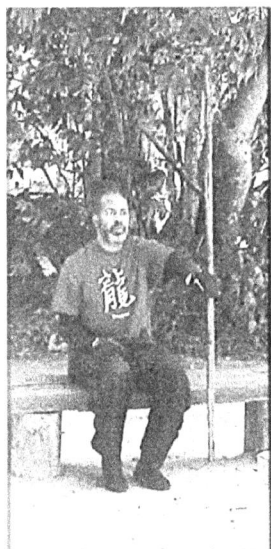

### #4

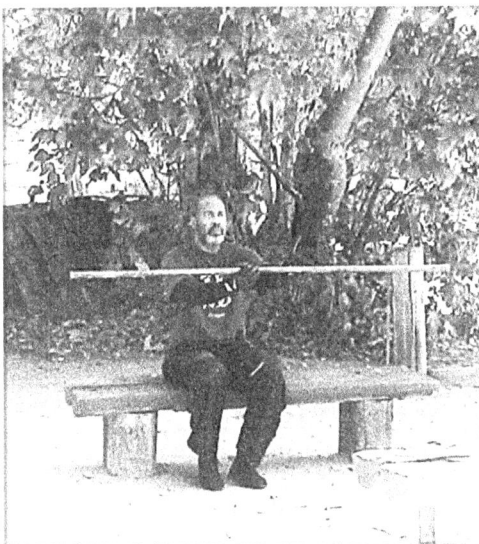

# #4 Lift each leg slowly from a seated position.

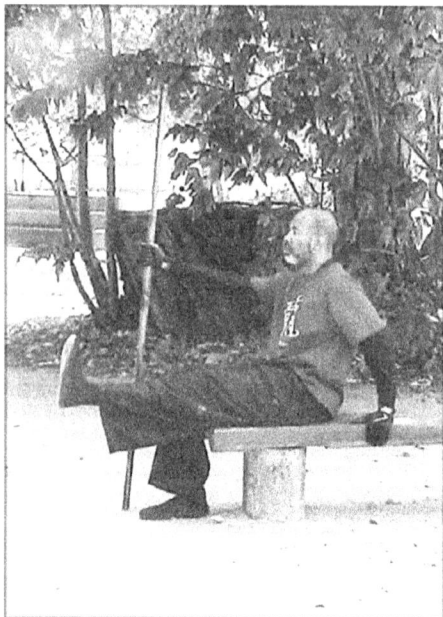

#1 Left Leg

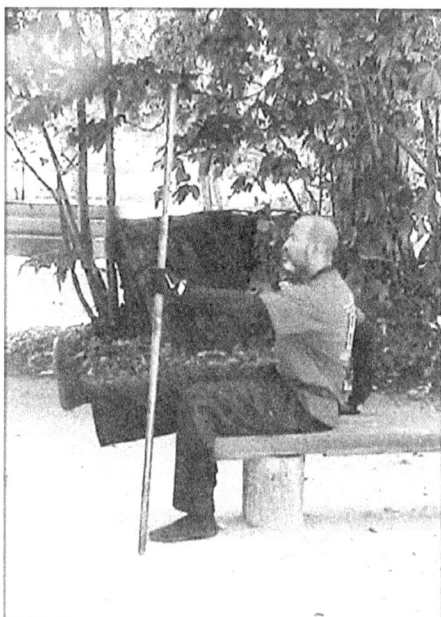

#2 Right Leg

# #5 Rotate your head, and upper body to the left, and right.

## #1 Right Side
## #2 Left Side

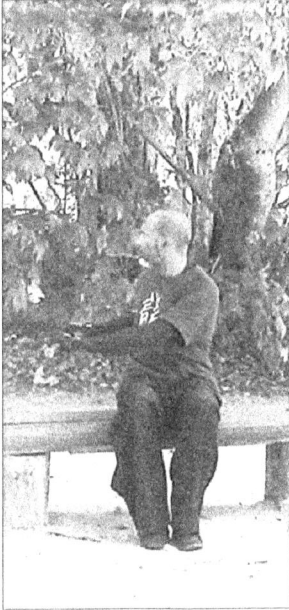
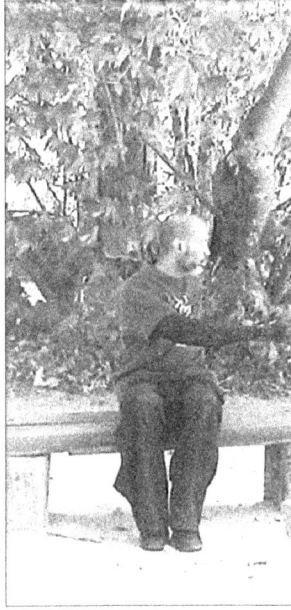

## Range of Motion Examples
*Pg. 162 - 169*

Give yourself a daily challenge, or goal to reach. It can be something as simple as getting out of bed, or relearning how to take a step. As these are simple tasks for some, most of you will feel like idiots. Let it be known that not everyone can move, function, or maneuver on a daily basis. Even the most seasoned of athletes, work on the basics. You are no different than any of them.

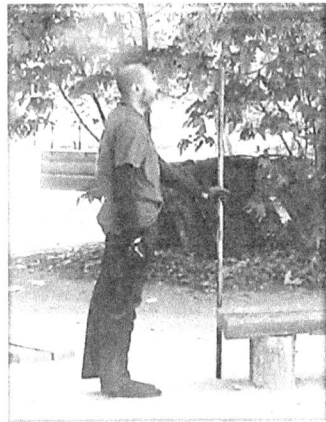

# ROM TEST
### (Continued)

## 1. Neck (Rotation)

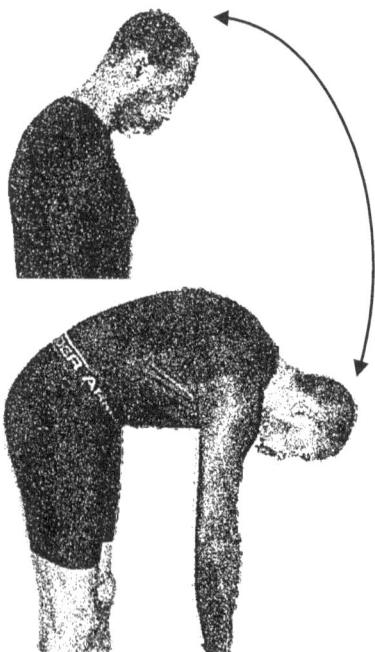

Rt.          Lt.

## 2. Back

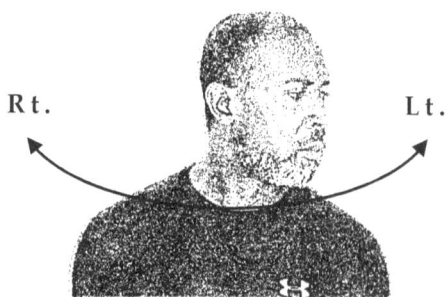

## 3. Lateral (Flexion)

Lt.        Rt.

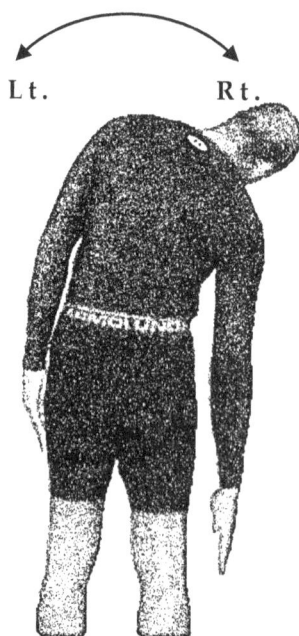

## 4. Neck

Back       Front

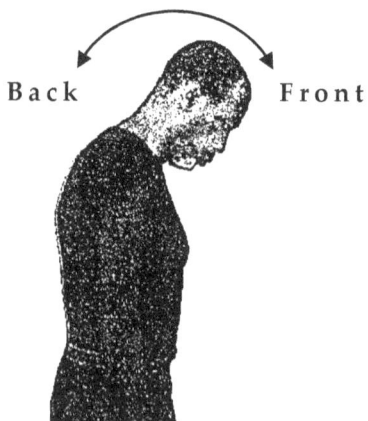

## 5. Neck (Lateral Bending)

Lt.        Rt.

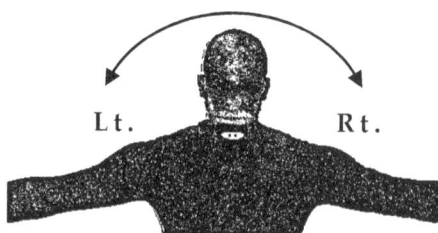

## 6. Knee (*Flexion*)

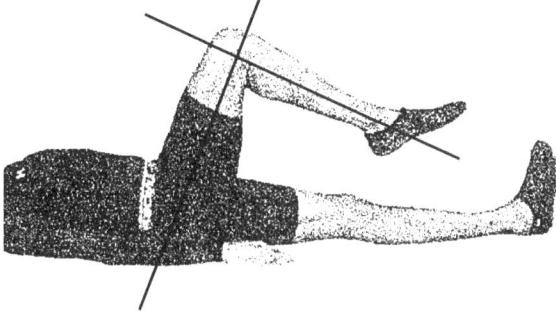

## 7. Hip (*Abduction*)

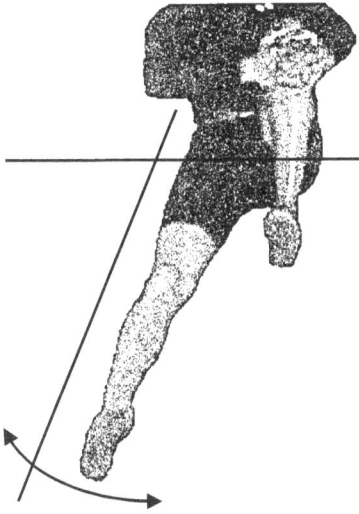

## 8. Hip (*Adduction*)

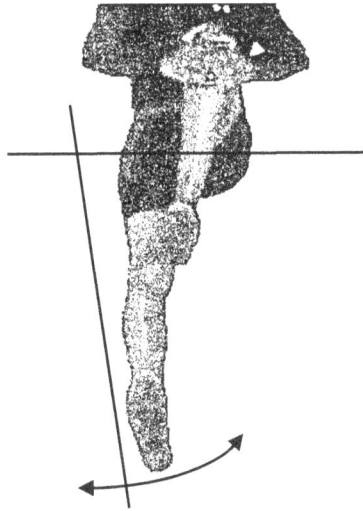

## 9. Hip (*Backward Extension*)

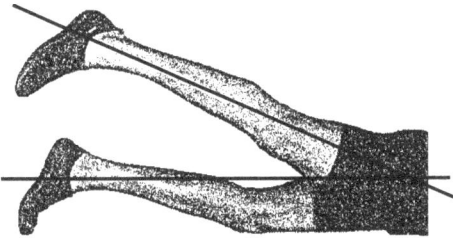

## 10. Hip (*Flexion*)

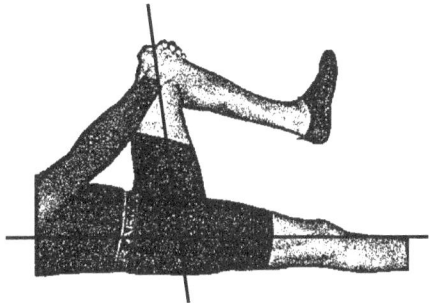

## 11. Elbow

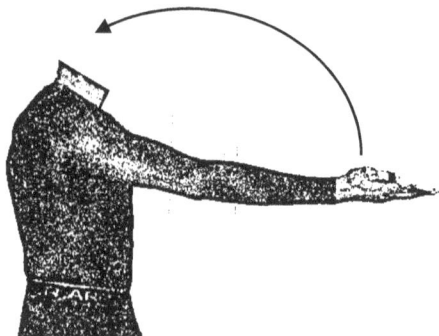

## 12. Shoulder (*Abduction - Adduction*)

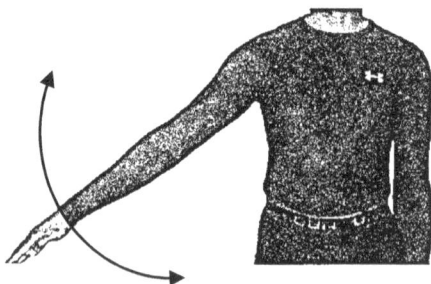

## 13. Shoulder (*Extension - Flexion*)

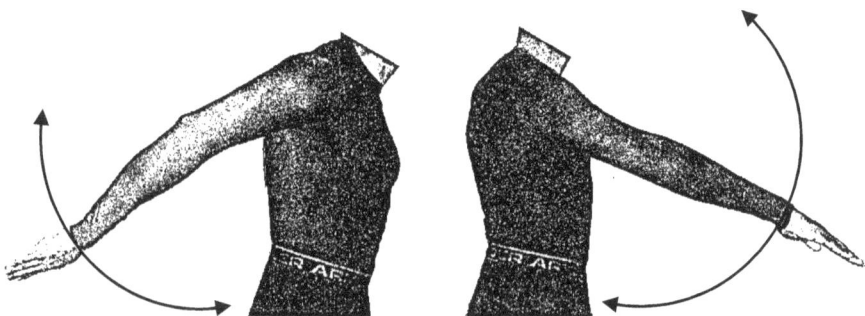

## 14. Forearm (*Pronation - Supination*)

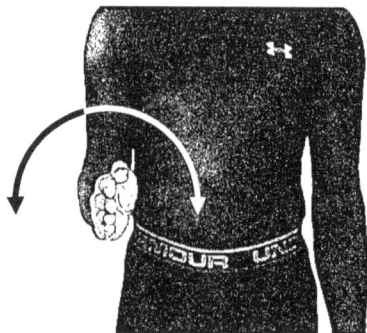

## 15. Ankle
*Left & Right*

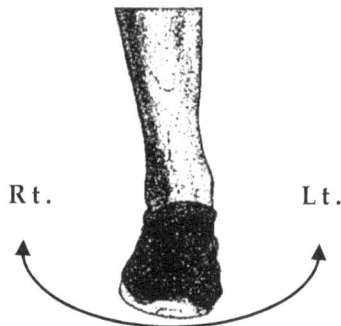

Rt.                                        Lt.

## 16. Ankle (*Flexion - Extension*)

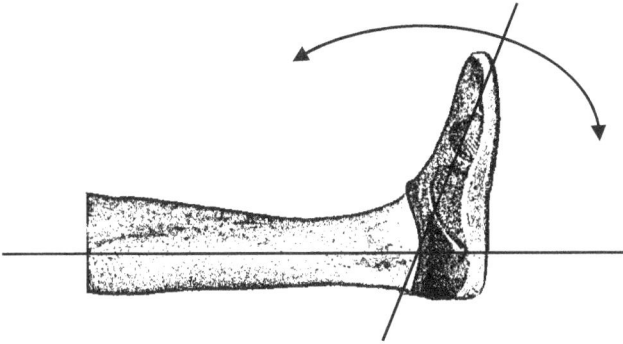

## 17. Wrist

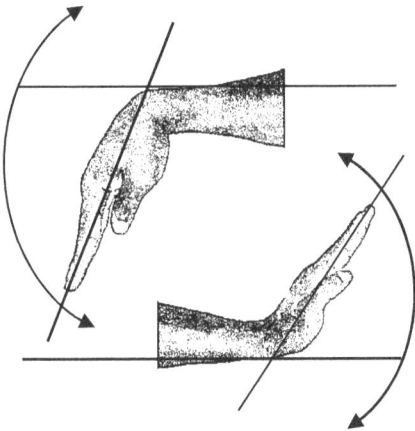

## 18. Wrist

*Radial*          *Ulnar*

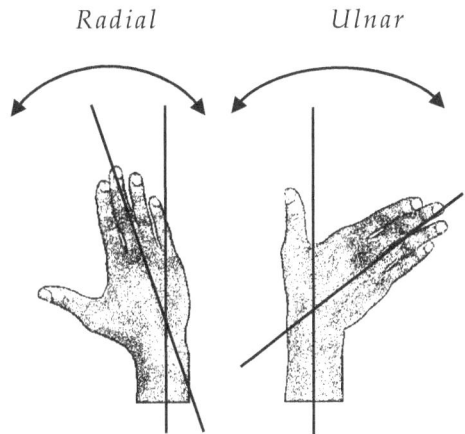

## 19. Thumb (*Mp Joint*)

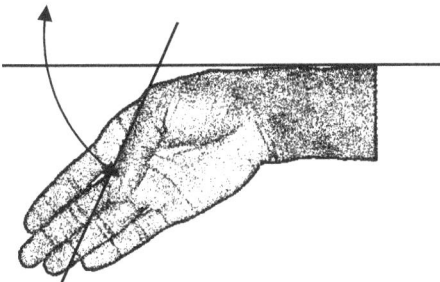

## 20. Thumb (*Ip Joint*)

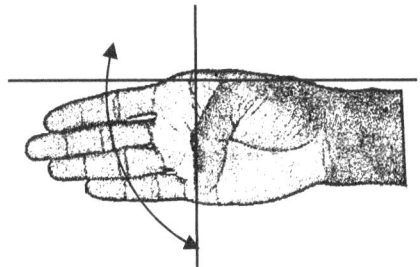

**Shoulder** *(Abduction - Adduction)*　　　**Knee** *(Flexion)*

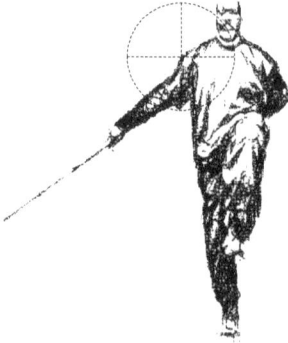

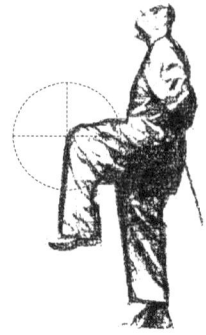

**Shoulder** *(Flexion - Extension)*　　　**Elbow** *(Extension)*

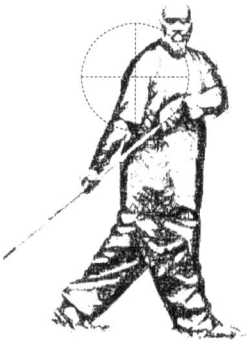

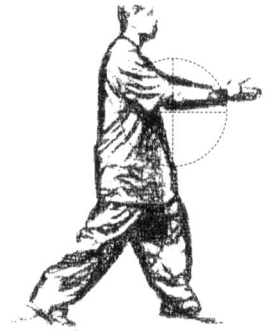

**Ankle** *(Flexion - Extension)*　　　**Hyperextension** *(Neck)*

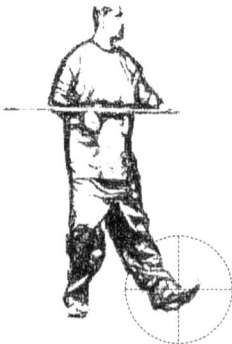

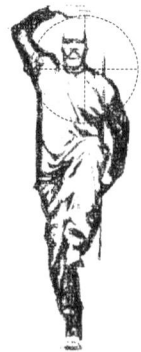

ROM  Exa. #1

**Neck** *(Rotation)*          **Back Extension**

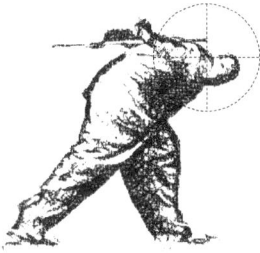

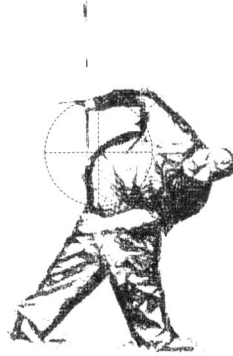

**Hip** *(Backward Extension)*      **Lateral** *(Extension)*

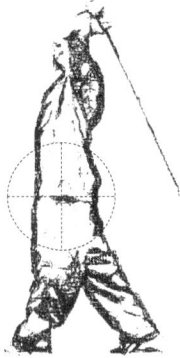

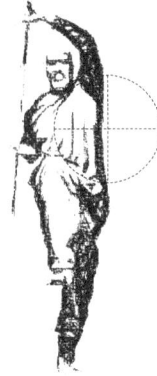

**Shoulder** *(Circumduction)*    **Hand** *(Pronation-Supination)*

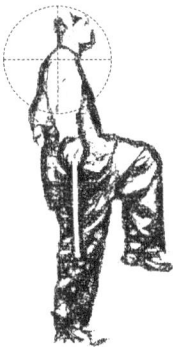

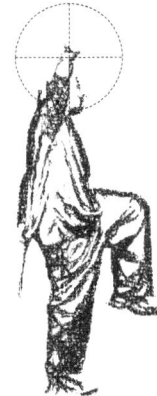

*ROM Exa. #2*

# Adduction

*Moving the upper limb towards the body. (**yin** - ☯)*

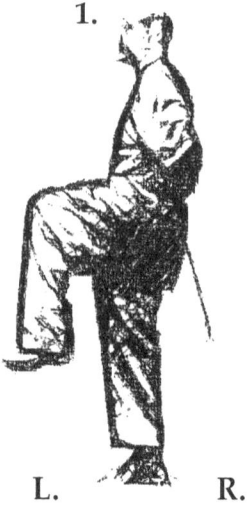

**1.**

**2.**

**Laterally**
*(sideways)*

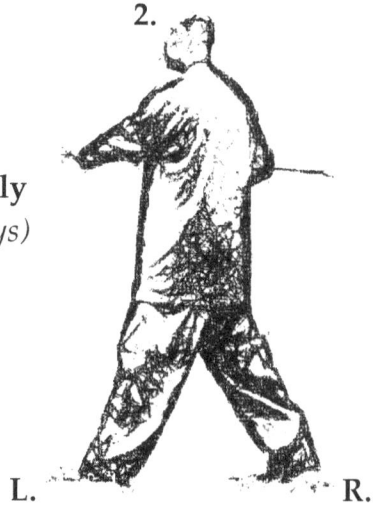

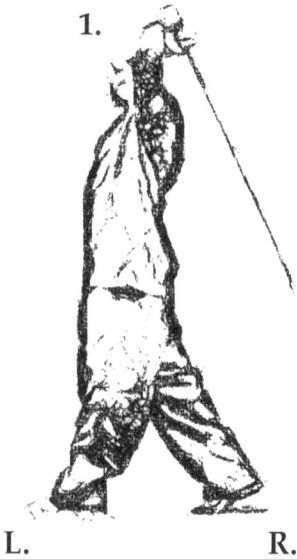

L.          R.          L.          R.

---

**1.**

**Anteriorly**
*(front)*

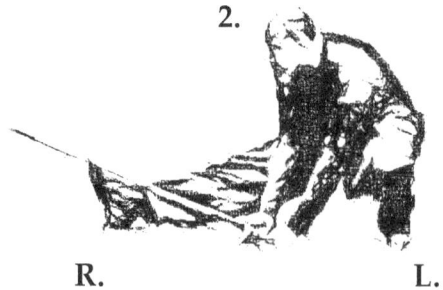

**2.**

L.          R.          R.          L.

# Abduction

*Moving the upper limb away from the body.* (**yang** - ☯)

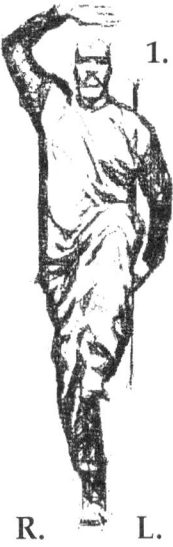

**1.**

**2.**

**Laterally**
*(sideways)*

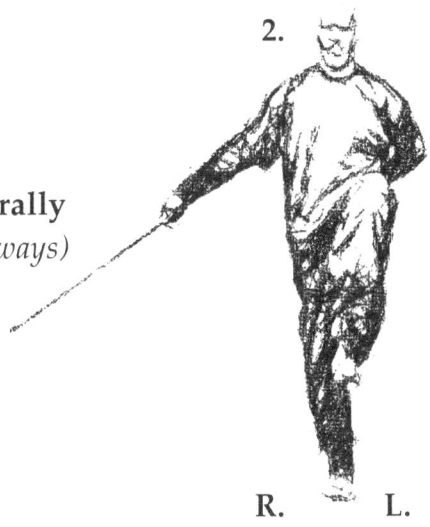

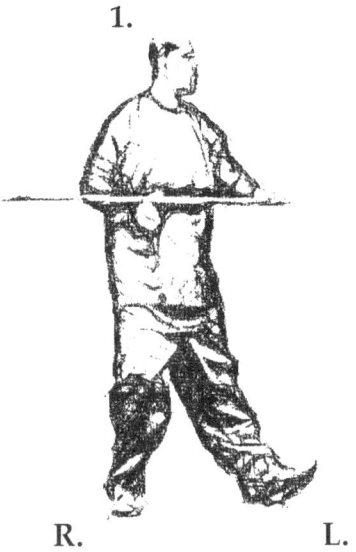

R.    L.

R.    L.

**1.**

**2.**

**Anteriorly**
*(front)*

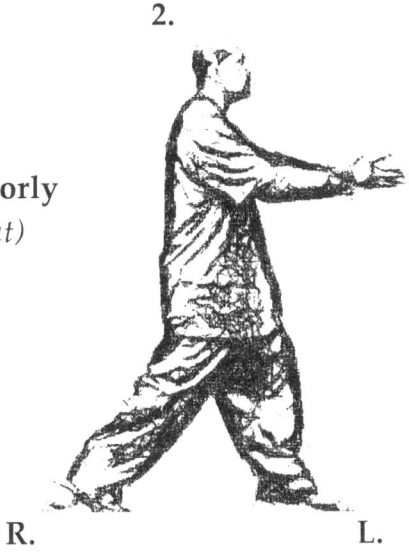

R.        L.

R.        L.

*Flexion* (Flexed)

**Yin** - *hard* = 🌑

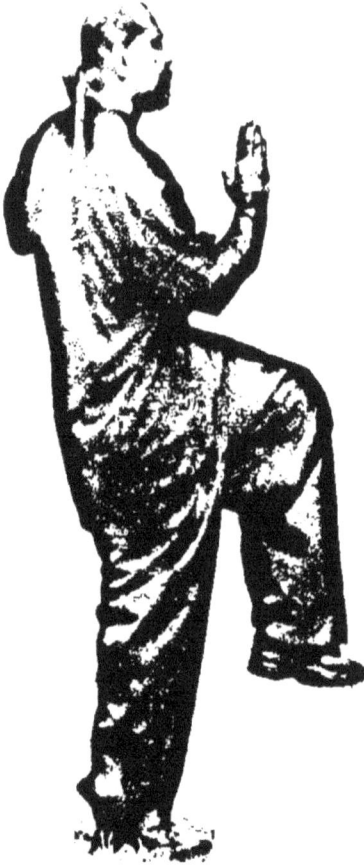

Flexion refers to the bending of a joint. Also to bring the upper and lower parts of a limb towards each other, or together. *Flexed* (r. & l. arm)

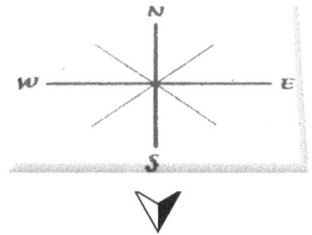

*yin*    ⬤    **L.**

*yang*    ◯    **R.**

#1     #2

**R.**    **L.**    **R.**    **L.**

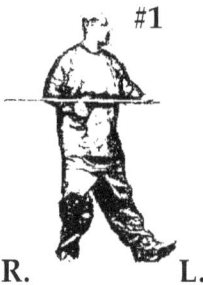

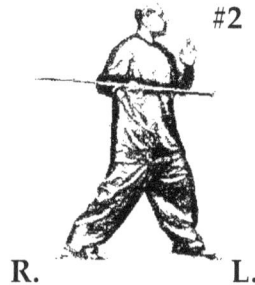

**Flexion**
*Exa. #1 & #2*
*yin*
🌑

## *Extension* (Extended)

**Yang** - *soft* =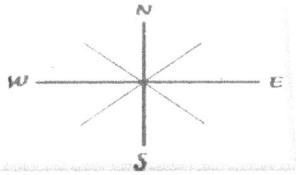

This is the reverse of the action. This results in the two parts of a limb moving away from each other, as opposed to bending inward. _Extended_ *(r. & l. arm).*

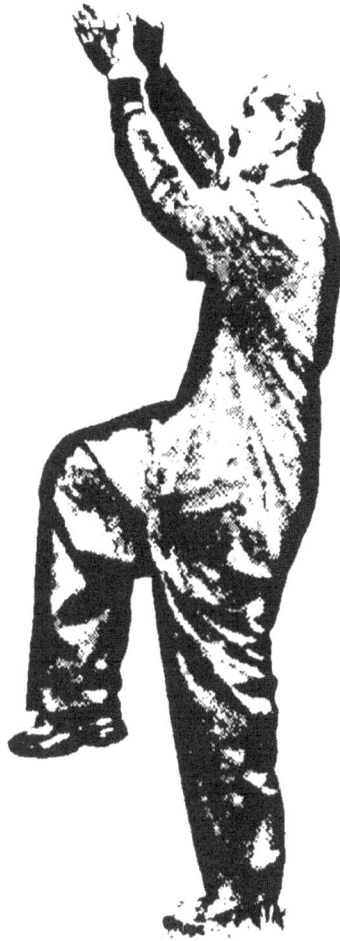

*yin* ⬭ R.

*yang* ⬭ L.

**Extension**
_Exa. #3 & #4_
*yang*

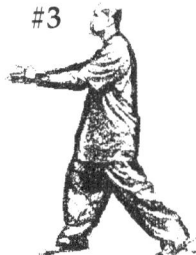

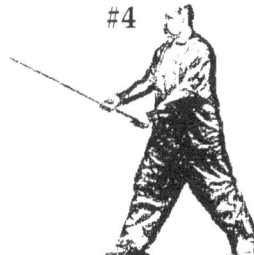

#3      #4

R.      L.      R.      L.

*Variance of Motion*

**#1 Lateral Motion** is the most natural and easiest to execute. However, to be most effective, you must learn to control both the rear and lead hand.

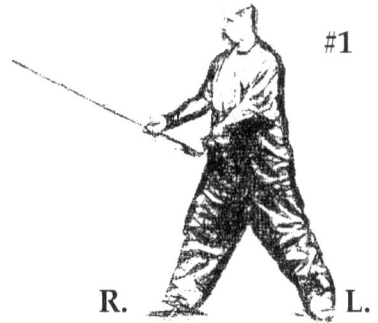

R.          L.

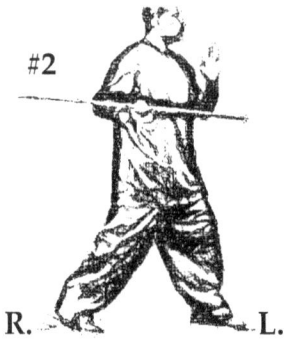

#2

R.          L.

**#2 Circular Motion** of which the hand moves from inside to outside, and vice versus. Should be executed with the emphasis on the contractions, and expansions of the arms.

**#3 Semicircular**, and **Diagonal Motions** have some advantages on specific areas, such as the arms. The latter are quite easy to execute.

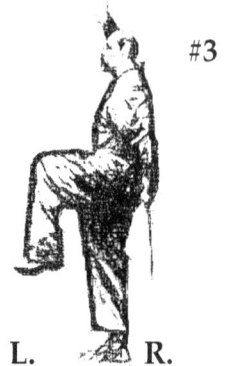

#3

L.          R.

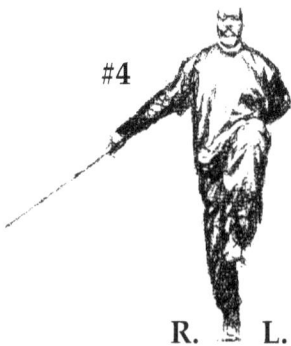

#4

R.   L.

**#4 Septime Motion** which is a diagonal action, can very often sweep into the inside line.

**Mechanics of Motion**

## 1st Class Lever

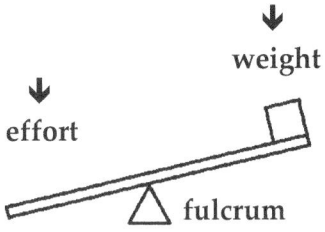

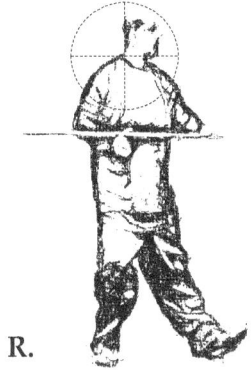

weight

effort

fulcrum

### Exa. #1
*The Neck*

R.      L.

## 2nd Class Lever

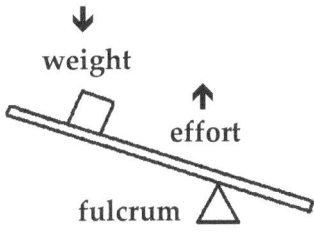

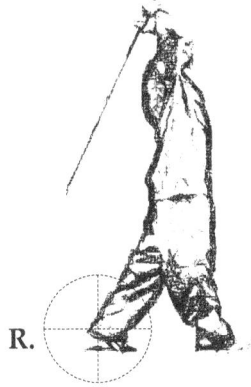

weight

effort

fulcrum

### Exa. #2
*The Rear Foot*

R.      L.

## 3rd Class Lever

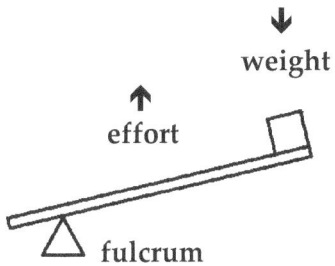

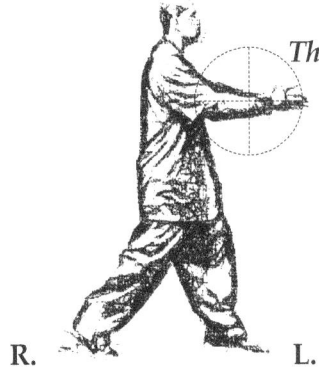

weight

effort

fulcrum

### Exa. #3
*The Lead Arm*

R.      L.

*Continued from pg. 151*

Over exercising weak muscles will only increase the weakness, and rob you of energy that you need for daily routines, or activities you enjoy. None of these exercises should cause you extreme pain. However, some discomfort is to be expected when tight muscles are stretched after a long hiatus. It is not a requirement for you to achieve full ROM on the first trial run, and should be something you work towards gradually. If you do experience severe pain when performing these exercises, stop. It may be that you are not executing the exercise correctly, or perhaps some modification should be done, so you can actively do the exercise.

Regular exercise contributes to a healthy body; therefore, immobility can have a negative effect. A joint that hasn't been worked sufficiently can begin to stiffen within 24 hours, and will eventually become inflexible. With overextended phases of immobility, the tendons and muscles can be affected. Some people exercise their joints naturally with normal activity, and daily living. Any time a joint cannot be worked in this fashion, the proponent should move it through regular exercise intervals to maintain muscle tone, and joint mobility. To help avoid strain, please try to remember to maintain your own body's active range of motion.

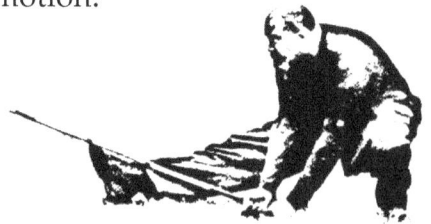

*The human body is a perfect machine. When using the stick or cane envision them as extensions, or parts of the latter. The goal is to find a perfect balance of mind, and body while in motion, as you breathe in, and out naturally, through each exercise segment.* (**Breath** = chi, or life force ).

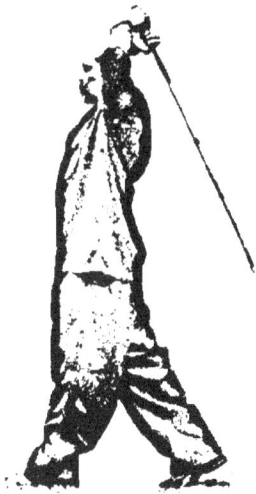

Whenever the advancement of a movement or motion is established, there must be a substantial effort to react, out of the intent. Our purpose is to advance, by gaining a vantage point. This is known as a responsive altercation. You must remain alert & fresh, by not prolonging or executing any motions, that exhaust the body or the mind.

YANG
*Substantial*

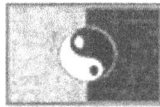

YIN
*Insubstantial*

As we examine this further, our form or function is to put the illness at a disadvantage, whereby we maintain control of it. Embrace it. Integrate each pose in its oneness, and then assimilate each, together as one being.

*The purest form should indicate its function by design. When measuring, guide by the mind, execute with the body. The mind moves the body, the body carries the soul.*

## Soul = spirit of vitality, or Shen

| | | |
|---|---|---|
| 1. ORGANIZE . . . . . . . . . . . . . . ? | *Tools* . . . . . . . . . . . .20% |
| 2. FAMILIARIZE . . . . . . . . . . . ? | *Knowing* . . . . . . . . 20% |
| 3. RATIONALIZE . . . . . . . . . . ? | *Realistic* . . . . . . . . . 20% |
| 4. MOBILIZE . . . . . . . . . . . . . ? | *Moving* . . . . . . . . . .20% |
| 5. ANALYZE . . . . . . . . . . . . . . ? | *Conditions* . . . . . . . .20% |

# Skeleton of The Human Body

*The Human Skeleton standing in,* **"The Ready Position."**

- *Skull*.........................

- *Neck*.........................
- *Clavicle*...................
- *Scapula*..............
- *Sternum*..............
- *Humerus*.............
- *Ribs*......................
- *Vertebral Column*....
- *Radius*...............
- *Ulna*.................
- *Pelvis*...............

**THE HAND**
- *Carpals*...........
- *Metacarpals*.....
- *Phalanges*........

- *Femur*...................

- *Patella*..............

- *Tibia*...................

- *Fibula*................

- *Tarsals*................
- *Metatarsals*...........
- *Phalanges*.............

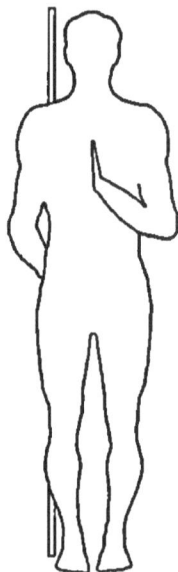

R. & L.

_____

**Light    Dark**

*yang        yin*

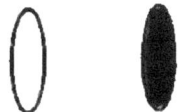

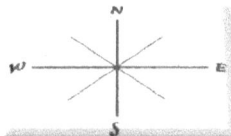

*South*

Friction is a force that opposes efforts to slide or roll one bone over another. There are no doubt numerous examples where we attempt to increase friction, as there are times that we try or attempt to decrease its effect. The amount of friction between one surface and another, depends upon the nature of the surfaces, and the forces pressing them together.

**Friction** #1 *The force of friction is parallel to the surface, which are sliding over each other, and opposite to the direction of motion.*

**Friction** #2 *It takes less force to keep something sliding, than it does to start it sliding.*

**Friction** #3 *At low speeds, friction usually decreases as speed increases; but at extremely fast speeds, friction increases tremendously.*

**Friction** #4 *Sliding friction is much less, than starting friction. Rolling friction is much less, than sliding friction.*

When an object rebounds from another object, it does so in a predictable manner. From these and other effects, you can calculate the speed of a motion. In the case of direction, you can determine the angular direction of the effort, and control the speed, of which friction is the driving force. The force, which acts on an object to distort it, is called stress. The distortion that occurs, is called strain, and is equal and proportional to the stress causing it.

*Exa. 1 - 4, show Joint Composition in* **"The Ready Position."**

# Shoulder & Hip Joints

### *Exa. 1* Ball & Socket

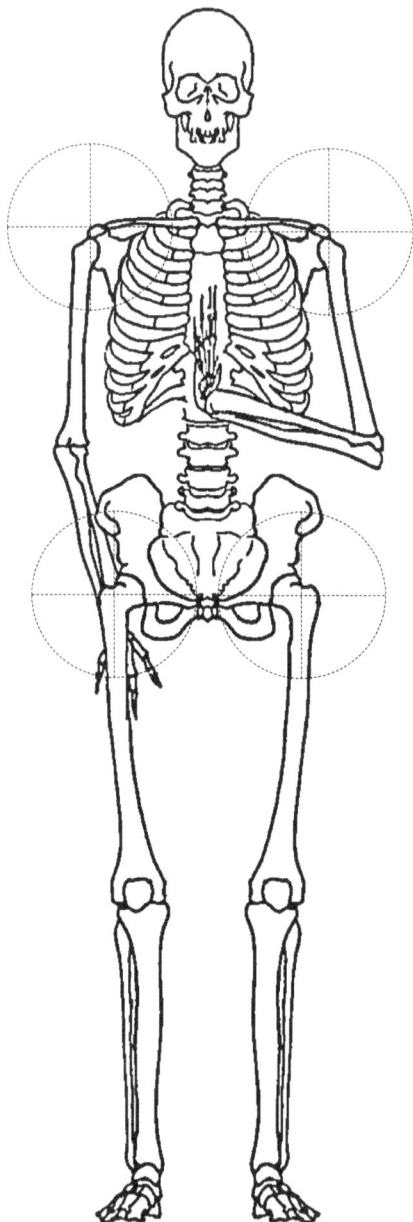

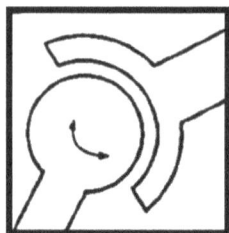

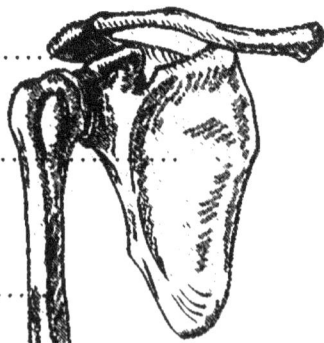

Clavicle......

Scapula.....

Humerus....

## Right Shoulder

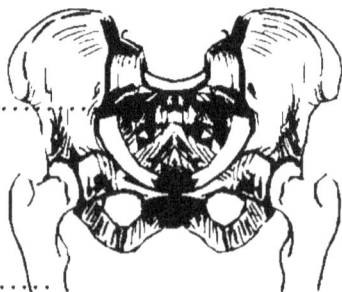

Pelvis.....

Femur......

## Pelvis

# *Elbow Joints*

## *Exa. II  Hinge & Pivot*

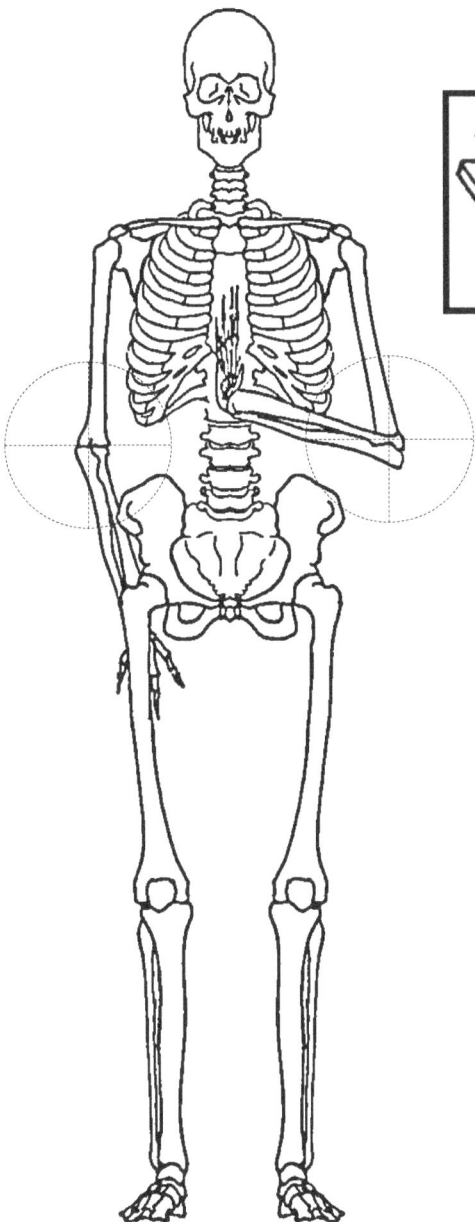

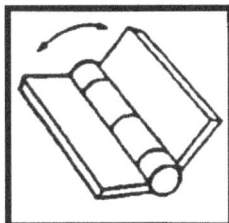
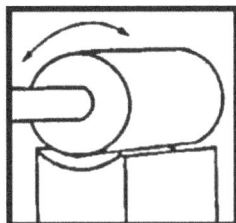

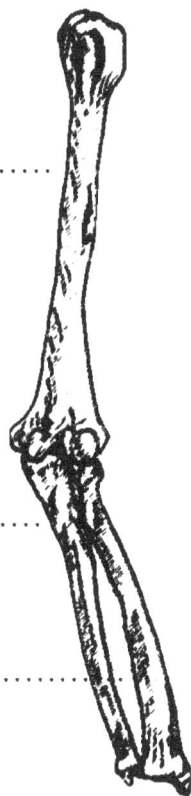

Humerus.......

Radius........

Ulna..............

## Right Elbow

# Knee Joints

*Exa. 111 Hinge*

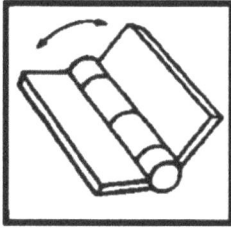

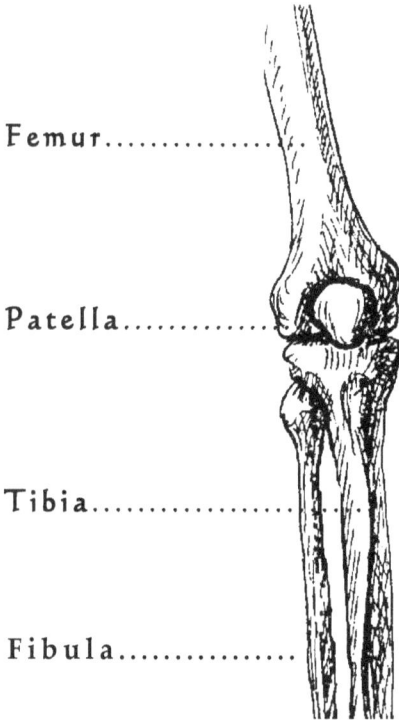

Femur..................

Patella..............

Tibia..................

Fibula...............

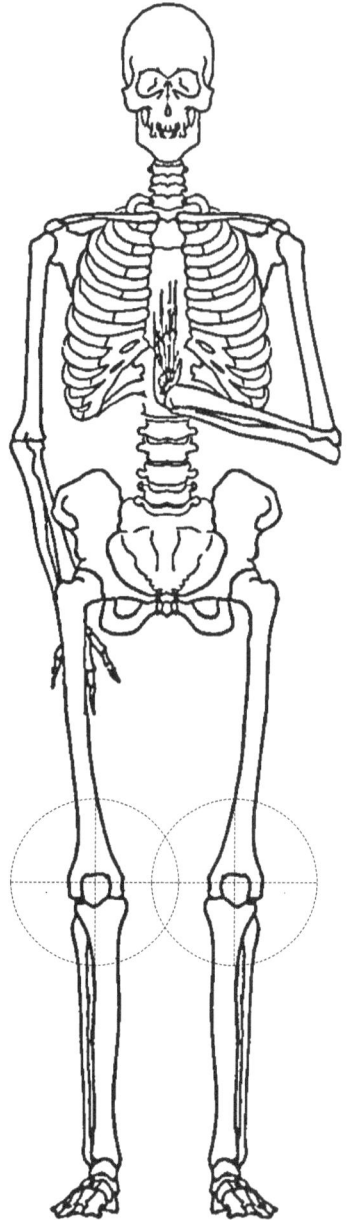

## Right Knee

# Foot & Ankle Joints

## Exa. IV Gliding

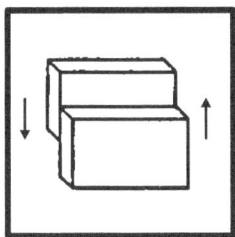

Hallux..................

Phalanges.........

Metatarsal.......
2$^{nd}$...............
3$^{rd}$...............
4$^{th}$...............
5$^{th}$...............

Cuneiform......
1$^{st}$ 2$^{nd}$ 3$^{rd}$...........
Cuboid.............

Navicular.........

Talus..............

Calcaneus.........

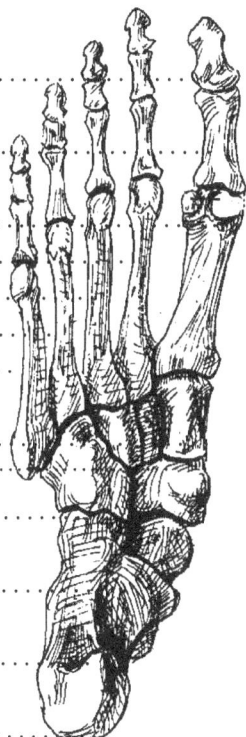

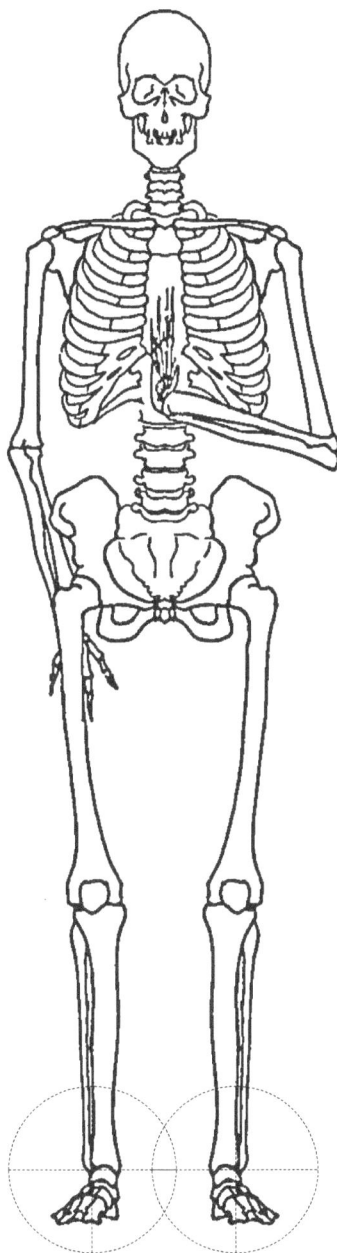

**Bottom of Right Foot**

# Synovial Joints I

## Ellipsoidal Joint

The Condyloid Joint or (Ellipsoid) - the joint of the _wrist_, consisting of a concave, and convexed system. This joint fits together in an odd shape allowing flexion, extension, abduction, and adduction movements.

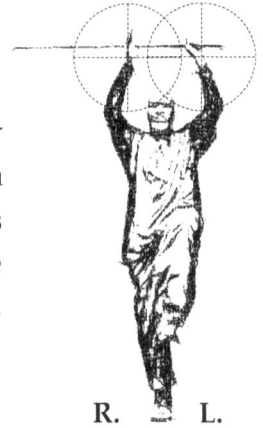

R.　L.

## Pivot Joint

The Pivot Joints - joints that allow rotation of external and internal movements. Movements that involve pronation or supination of the _hand_ or _forearm_ where one bone rotates about another.

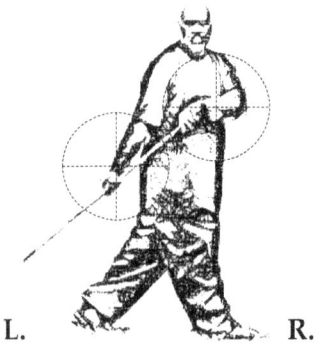

L.　R.

## Gliding Joint

The Plane Joint or Gliding Joint - found in the _wrist_ or _ankle_, these joints allow gliding or sliding movement. These joints are flat or almost flat about the surface area. Movement is tight.

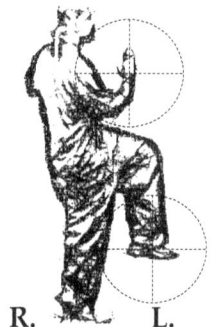

R.　L.

# Synovial Joints II

## Saddle Joint

The Saddle Joint - similar to the condyloid joint, but with the exception of axial rotation. Such joints are biaxial and relate to the **thumbs**. In the saddle joint the opposing surfaces are reciprocally concave-convex.

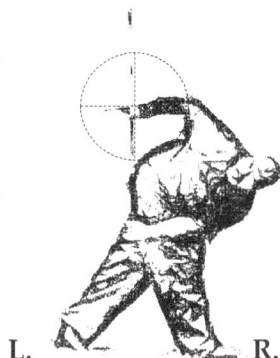

L.          R.

## Hinge Joint

The Hinge Joints - joints that are local to the **knee** and **elbow** only. Shaped like the hinge on a door, the connecting bones opens to 180 degrees. Able to create obtuse, and acute angles.

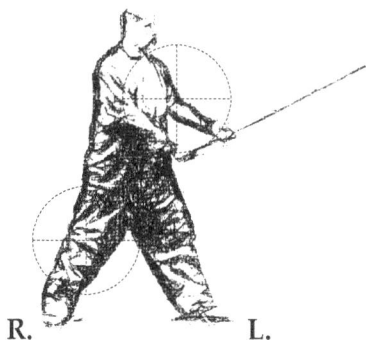

R.          L.

## Ball & Socket Joint

The Ball & Socket Joint - able of moving in almost any direction, this joint is local to the **shoulder** and **hip** area. The ball shaped surface of one rounded bone fits into the cup-like depression of another bone.

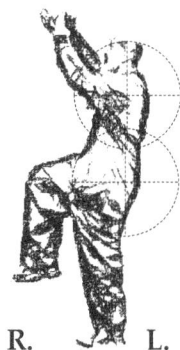

R.          L.

# The Ready Position pt. III
## Muscles & Parts of the Human Body

A & Ω

Right Brain . . . . . . . . . . . . . . . . . . . . . . . . Left Brain
Staff . . . . . . . . . . . . . . . . . . . . . . . . . . . . . Head
Right Side of Neck . . . . . . . . . . . . . . Left Side of Neck
Right Shoulder. . . . . . . . . . . . . . . . . Left Shoulder
Right Deltoid . . . . . *Left Hand* . . . . . . Left Deltoid
Right Triceps . . . . . . . . . . . . . . . . . Left Triceps
Right Bicep . . . . . . . . . . . . . . . . . . Left Bicep
Right Elbow . . . . . . . . . . . . . . . . . .Left Elbow
Right Forearm . . . . . . *Stomach* . . . . . .Left Forearm
Right Abdominal . . . . . . . . . . . . . . . Left Abdominal
Tan Tien . . . . . . . . . . . . . . . . . . . . . Tan Tien
Right Hip . . . . . . . . . . . . . . . . . . . . .Left Hip
Right Thigh . . . . . . . . . . . . . . . . . . .Left Thigh
Right Quadriceps . . . . . . . . . . . . .Left Quadriceps
Right Leg . . . . . . . . . . . . . . . . . . . . Left Leg
Right Knee . . . . . . . . . . . . . . . . . . Left knee
Right Calf . . . . . . . . . . . . . . . . . . . .Left Calf
Right Shin Bone . . . . . . . . . . . . . . Left Shin Bone
Right Ankle . . . . . . . . . . . . . . . . . .Left Ankle
Right Instep . . . . . . . . . . . . . . . . . Left Instep
Right Foot . . . . . . . . . . . . . . . . . . . Left Foot

*In the following examples, study the ROM in each exercise. Also, note the different parts of the body that receive work.*

**A gracious bird, salutes the Heavens.** (*exa.1*)
**A poignant bird, embraces the new day.** (*exa.2*)
*Exam. #1 - #20 show The Purest using, **The Bamboo Stick**, 48" long.*

*A~ROM*

*Example~1*

*The*

*Salute*

*Left Side*

*yin*

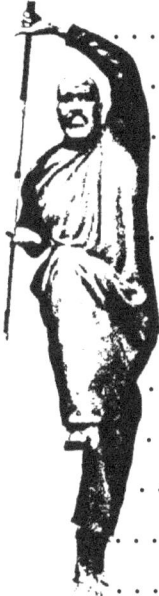

. . . . . . . . . . . . . . . . Left Forearm
. . . . . . . . . . . . . . . Left Triceps
. . . . . . . . . . . . . . Left Deltoids
. . . . . . . Left Latissimus Dorci
. . . . . . . . . . . . . . . . . Stomach
. . . . . . . . . . . Left Abdominal
. . . . . . . . . . . . . . . . Left Hip
. . . . . . . . . . . . . . . Right Leg
. . . . . . . . . . . . . . . . Left Leg
. . . . . . . . . . . . . . . . Left Calf
. . . . . . . . . . . . . . Left Instep
. . . . . . . . . . . . . . . Left Foot

Right Forearm . . . . . . . . . . . . . .
Right Triceps . . . . . . . . . . . . .
Right Deltoids. . . . . . . . . . . . .
Right Latissimus Dorci . . . . . . . .
Stomach . . . . . . . . . . . . . . . . .
Right Abdominal. . . . . . . . . . . .
Right Hip . . . . . . . . . . . . . . . .
Left Leg . . . . . . . . . . . . . . . . .
Right Leg. . . . . . . . . . . . . . . . .
Right Calf . . . . . . . . . . . . . . . .
Right Instep . . . . . . . . . . . . . . .
Right Foot . . . . . . . . . . . . . . . .

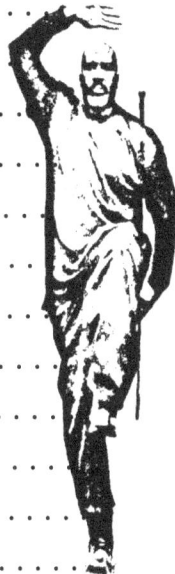

*A~ROM*

*Example~2*

*The*

*Embrace*

*Right Side*

*yang*

# Example - 3
## A-ROM, (Exa. 1 - 3)

| | Yang | Yin |
|---|---|---|
| #1 Insightful Crane, sweeps to the south. | | |
| #2 Secure the right wing. | r. | l. |
| #3 Crane spreads his right wing open. | | |

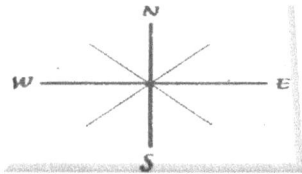

Your weight is distributed on your right leg, throughout the exercises.

| Right Side | Left Side |
|---|---|
| Shoulder | Shoulder |
| Deltoid | Deltoid |
| Biceps | Biceps |
| Triceps | Triceps |
| Forearm | Forearm |
| Leg | Leg & Knee |
| Foot & Instep | Foot & Instep |

# Example - 4
## A-ROM, (Exa. 4 - 6)

| #4 Secure the left wing. | Yang | Yin |
|---|---|---|
| |  |  |
| #5 Crane spreads his left wing open. | r. | l. |
| #6 Powerful bird, holds up the sky. | 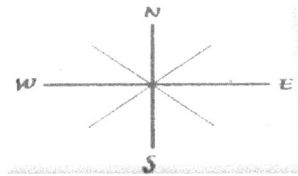 | |

Your weight is distributed on your right leg, throughout the exercises.

| Right Side | Left Side |
|---|---|
| Shoulder | Shoulder |
| Deltoid | Deltoid |
| Biceps | Biceps |
| Triceps & Lats. D. | Triceps & Lats. D. |
| Forearm | Forearm |
| Leg | Leg & Knee |
| Foot & Instep | Foot & Instep |

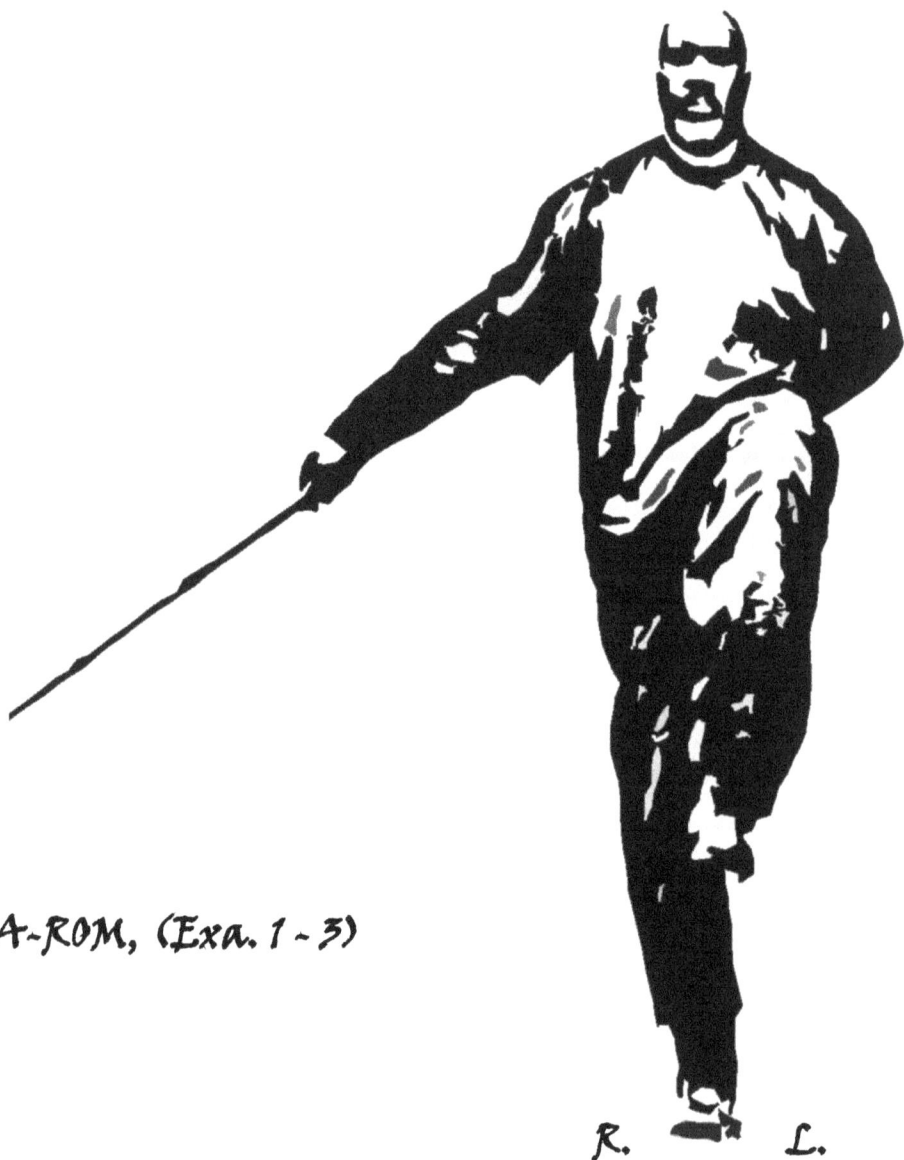

*Example - 3 continued*

**A-ROM, (Exa. 1 - 3)**

R.      L.

# Example - 4 continued

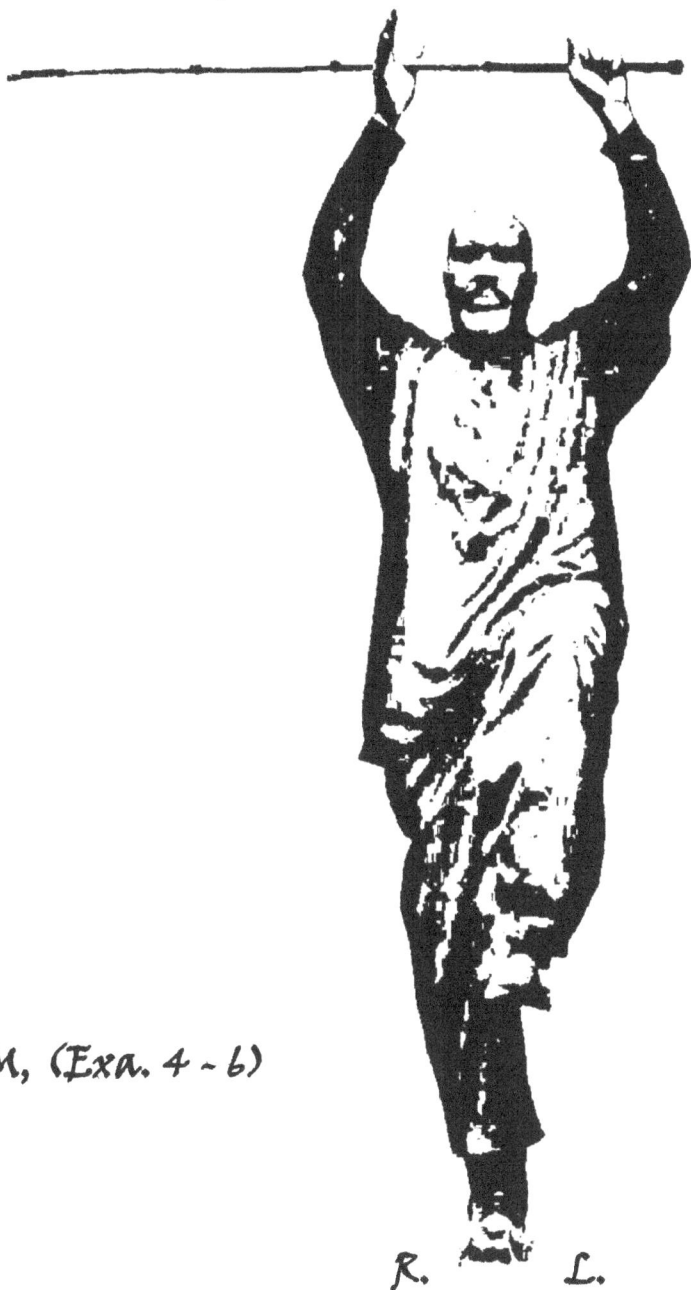

A-ROM, (Exa. 4 - 6)

R.    L.

# A-ROM #7 Advance to release.
## (Exa. 5)

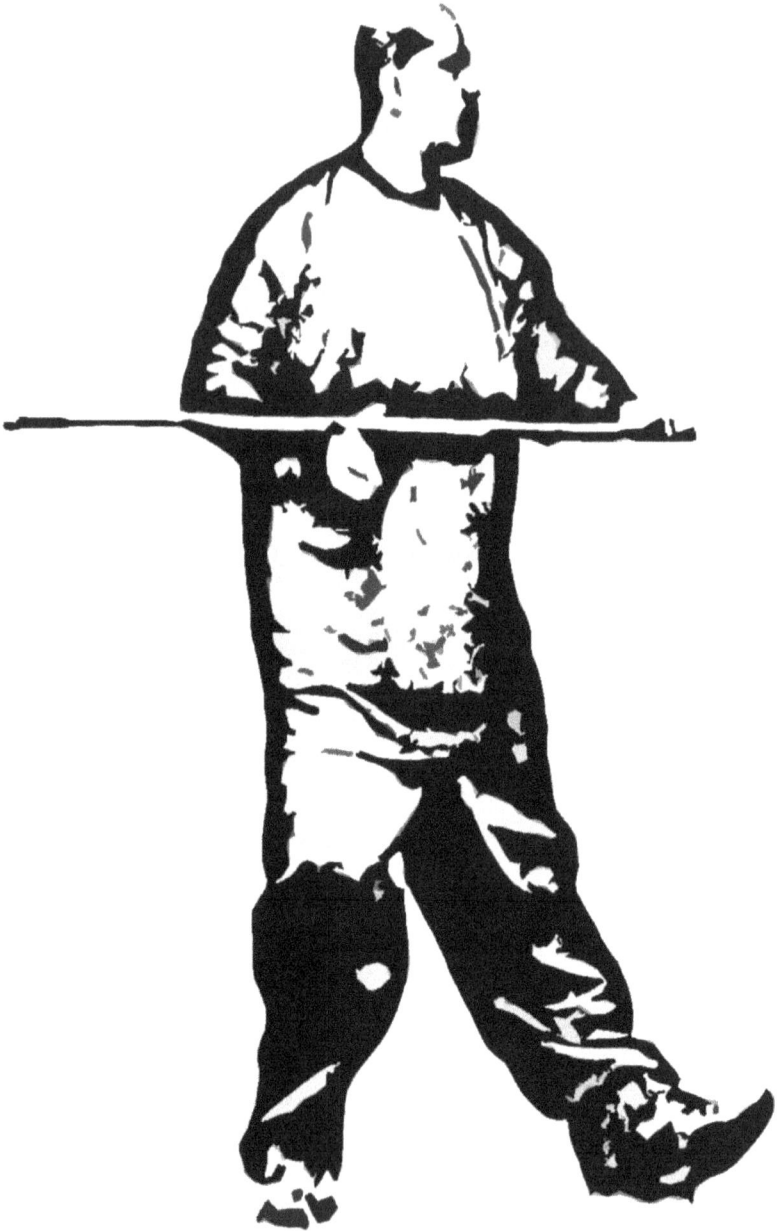

R.                                    L.

# A-ROM  #8 Immaculate bird strikes its prey.
## (Exa. 6)

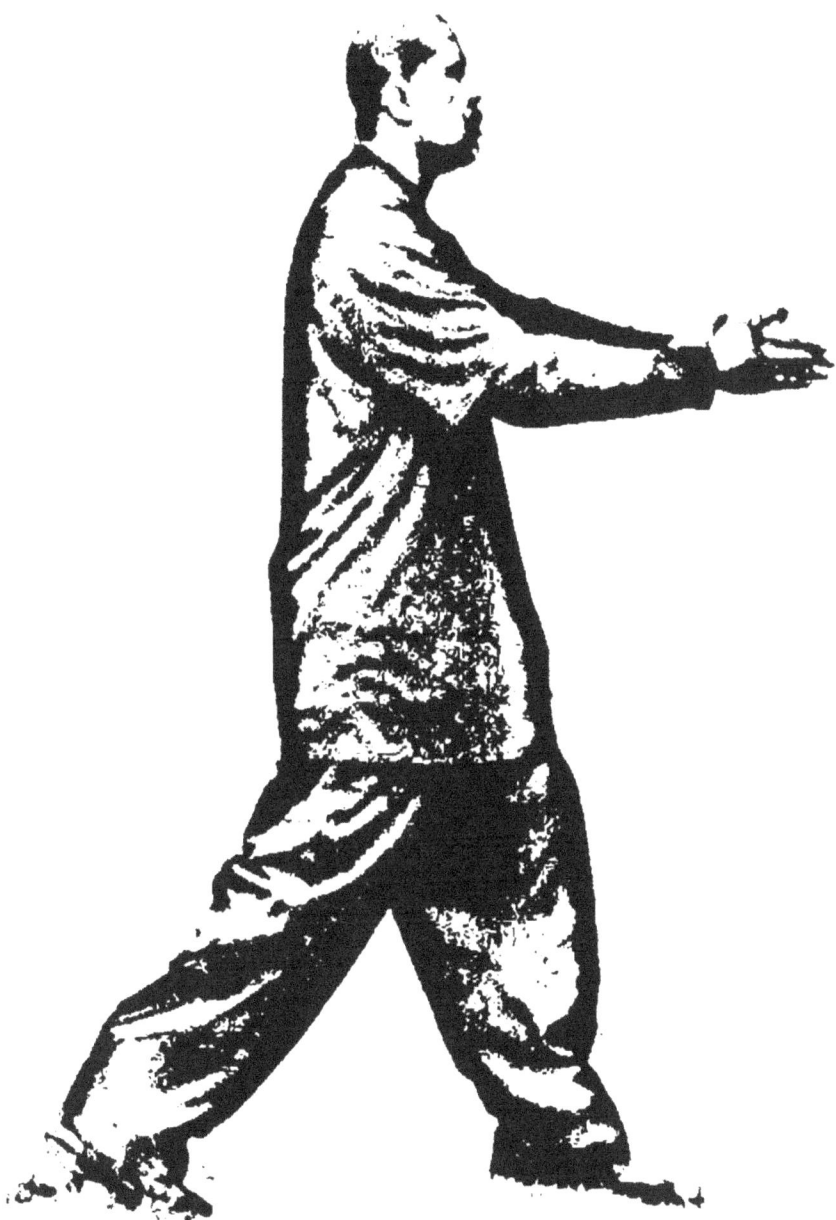

R.                                        L.

# A-ROM  #9 Diligent Crane rotates his beak.
## (Exa. 7)

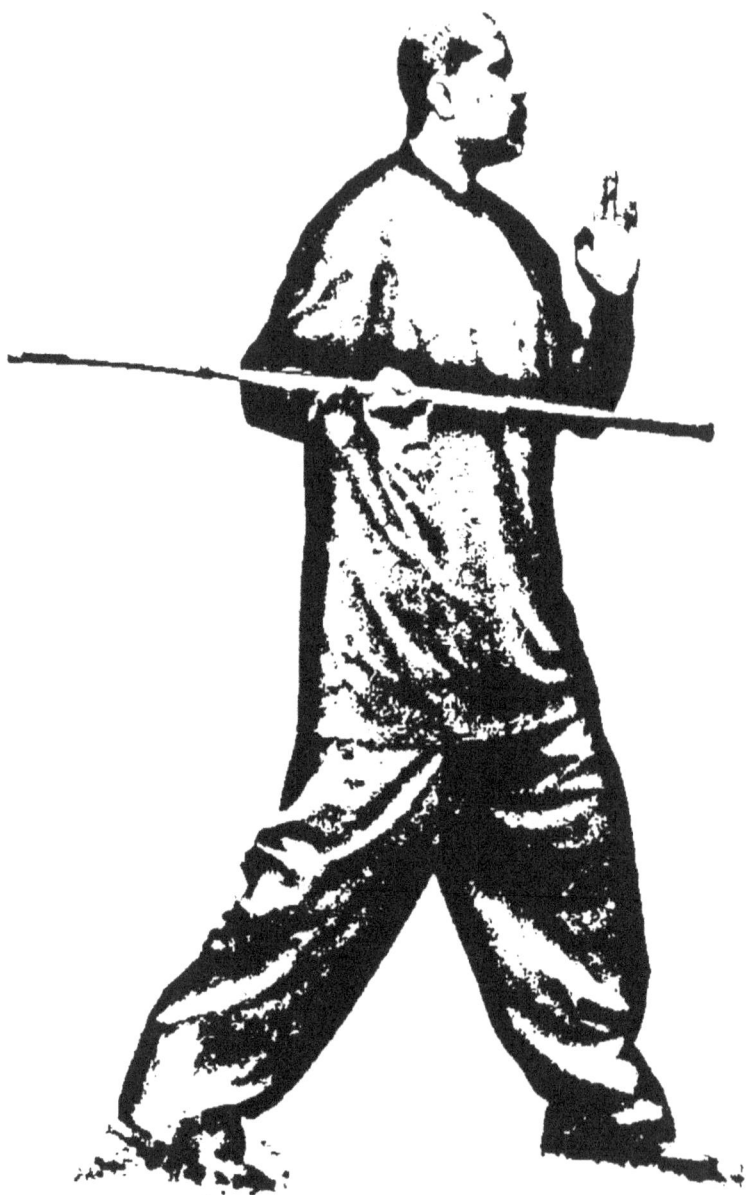

R.                                    L.

# A-ROM  #10 Divine bird looks to Heaven.
## (Exa. 8)

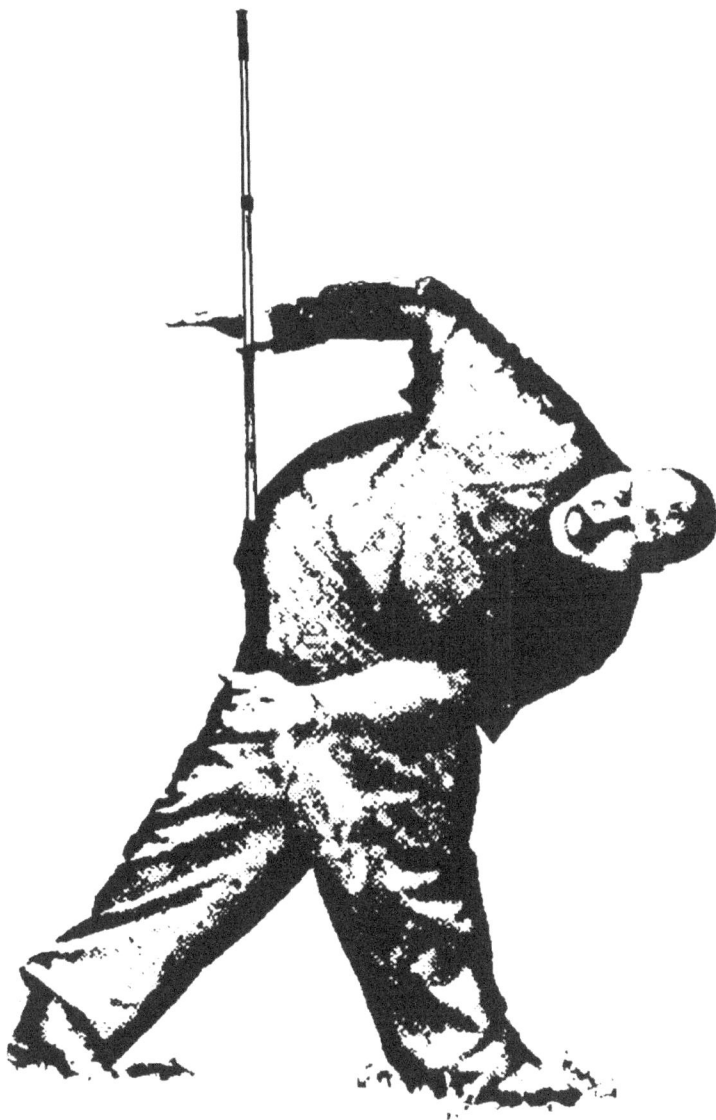

L.                                    R.

# A-ROM #11 Ambitious Crane looks for food.
## (Exa. 9)

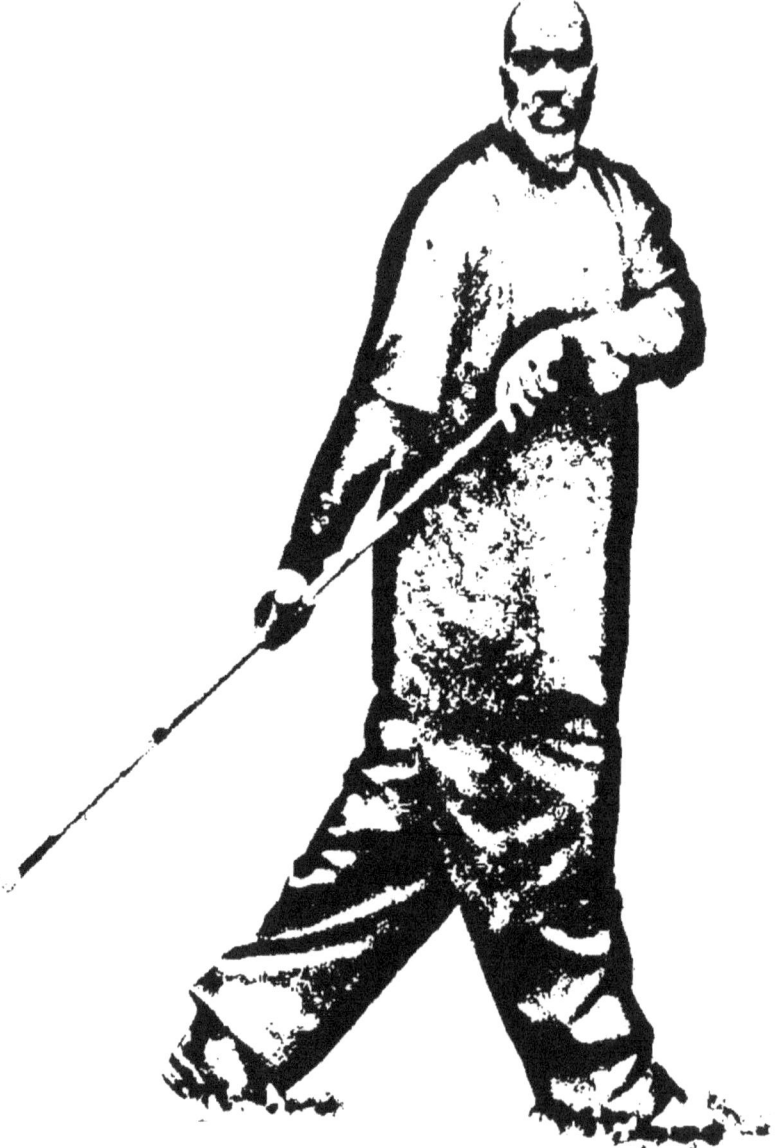

L.                    R.

# A-ROM  #12 Heroic bird stretches his wings.
## (Exa. 10)

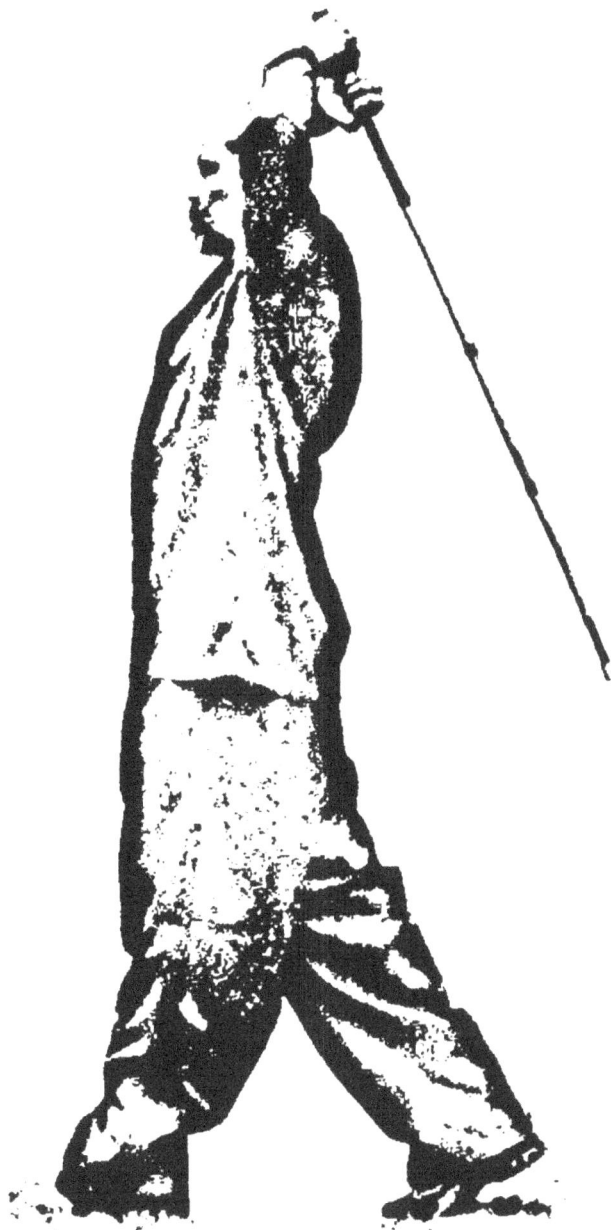

L.                    R.

# A-ROM  #13 Uncanny Crane stomps his foot.
## (Exa. 11)

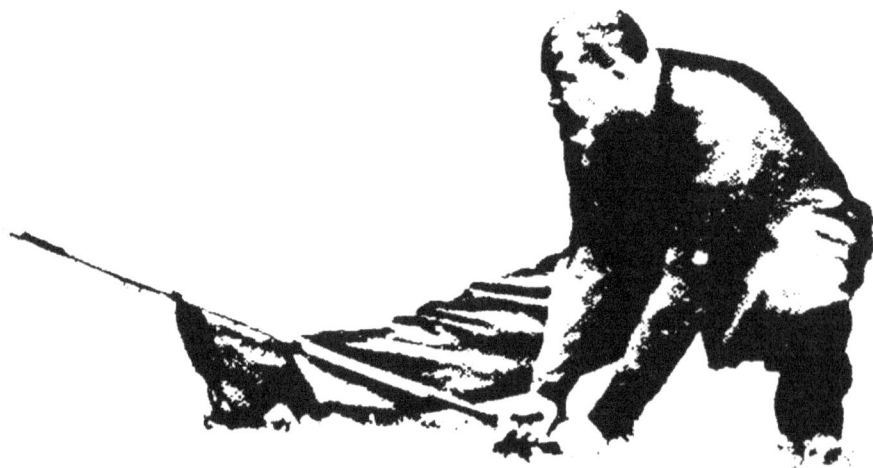

R.                                    L.

# A-ROM  #14 Fearless bird grabs a fish.
## (Exa. 12)

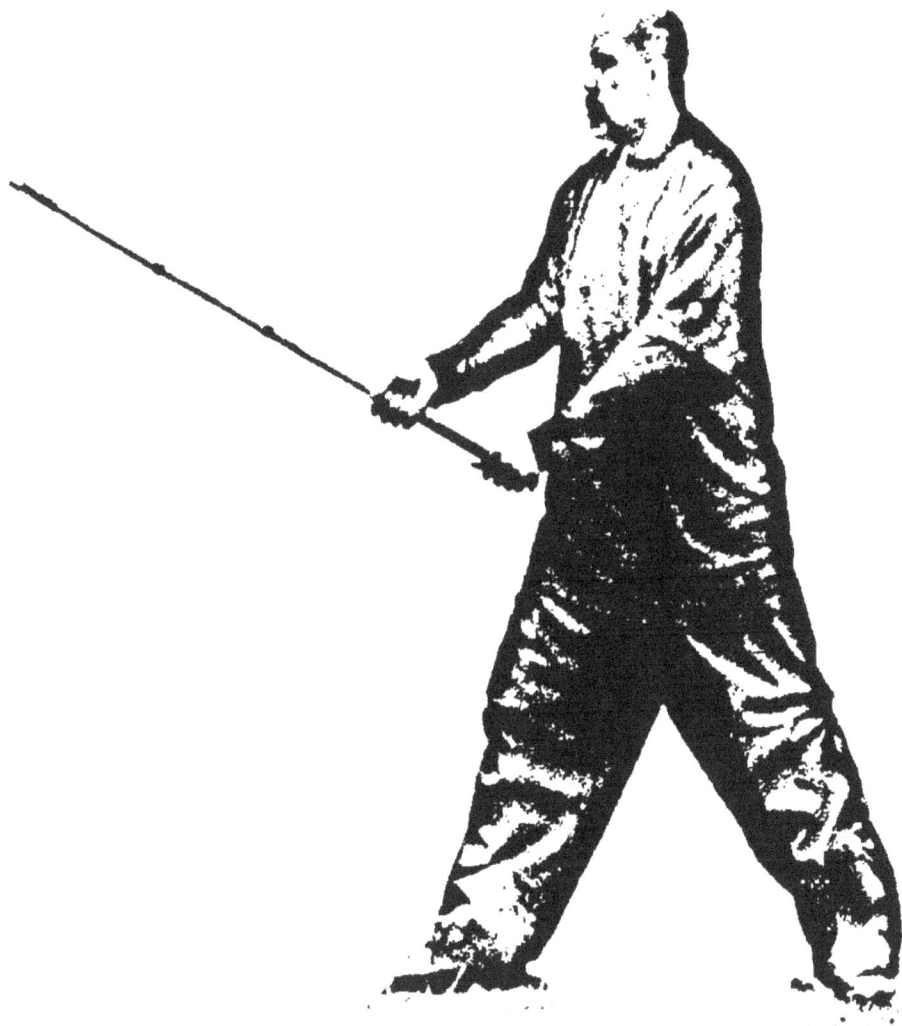

R.                          L.

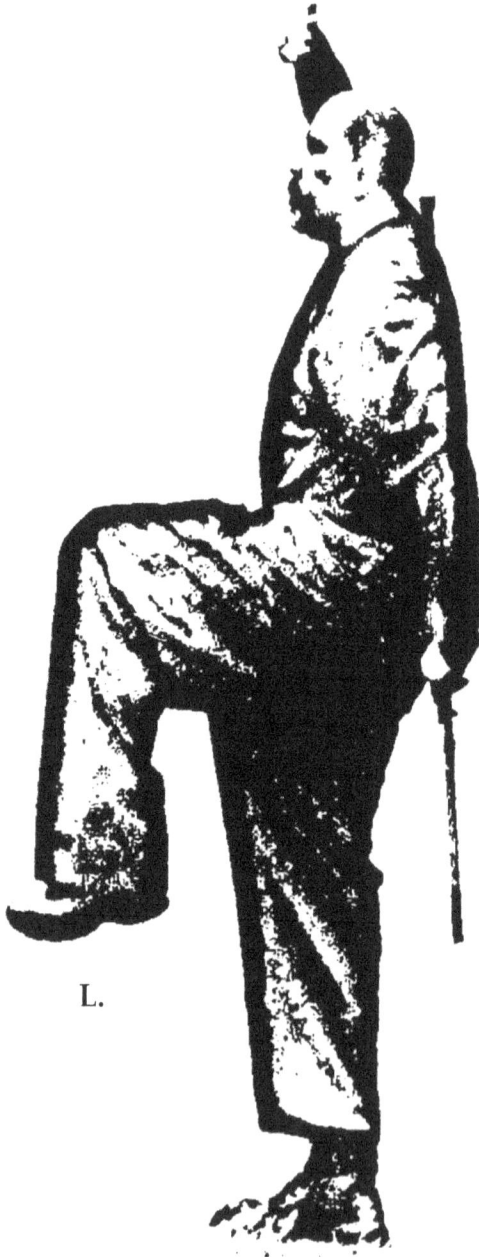

L.

R.

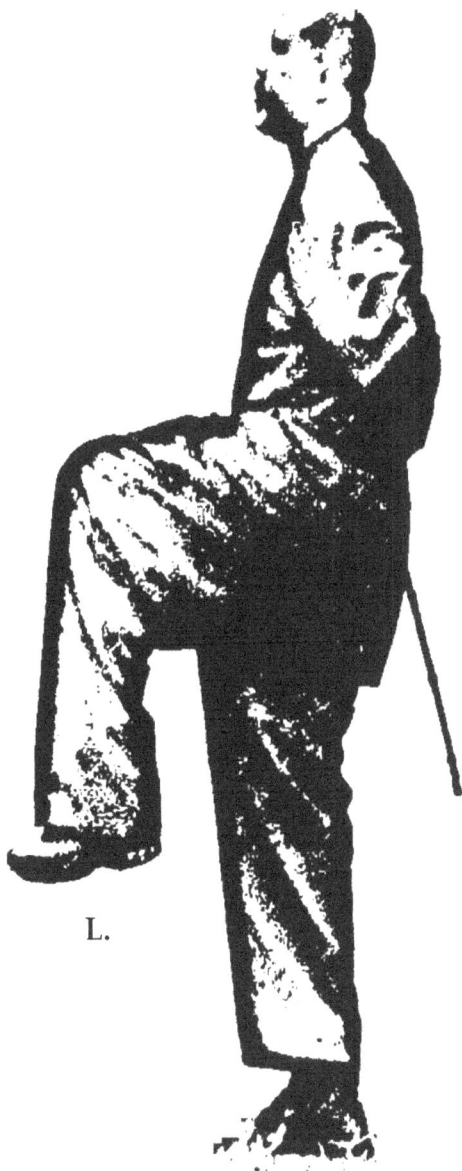

L.

R.

# A-ROM  #17(A.) Lofty bird goes down under.
## (Exa. 15)

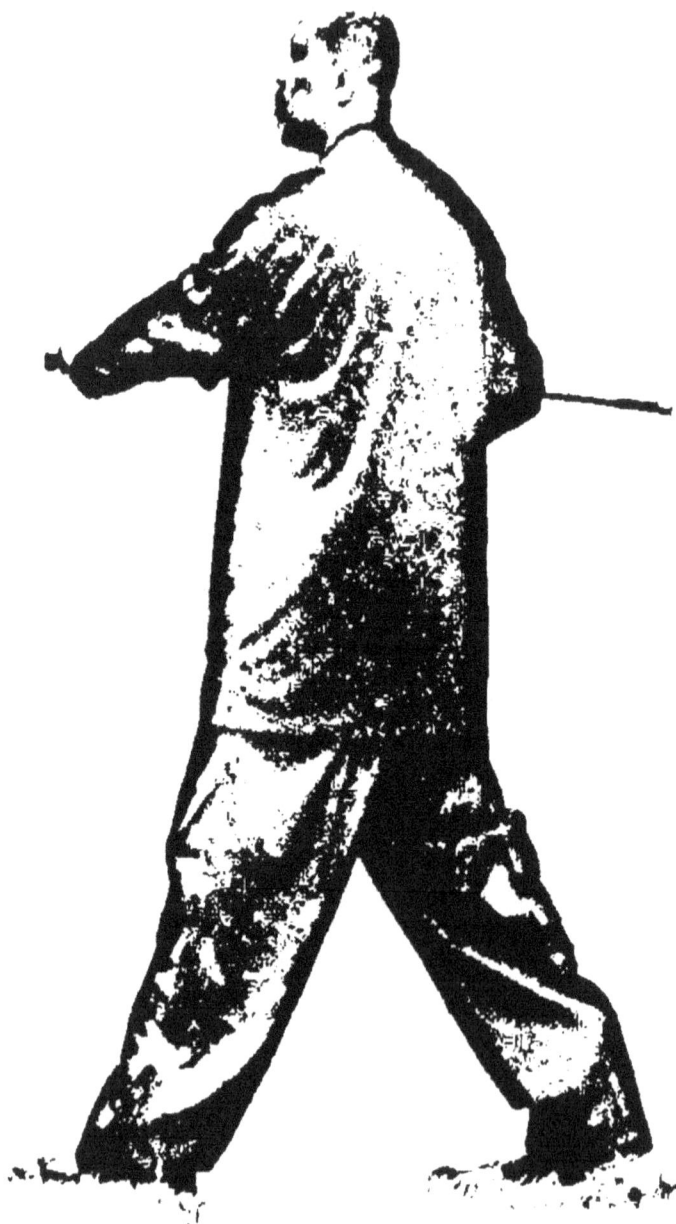

L.                                        R.

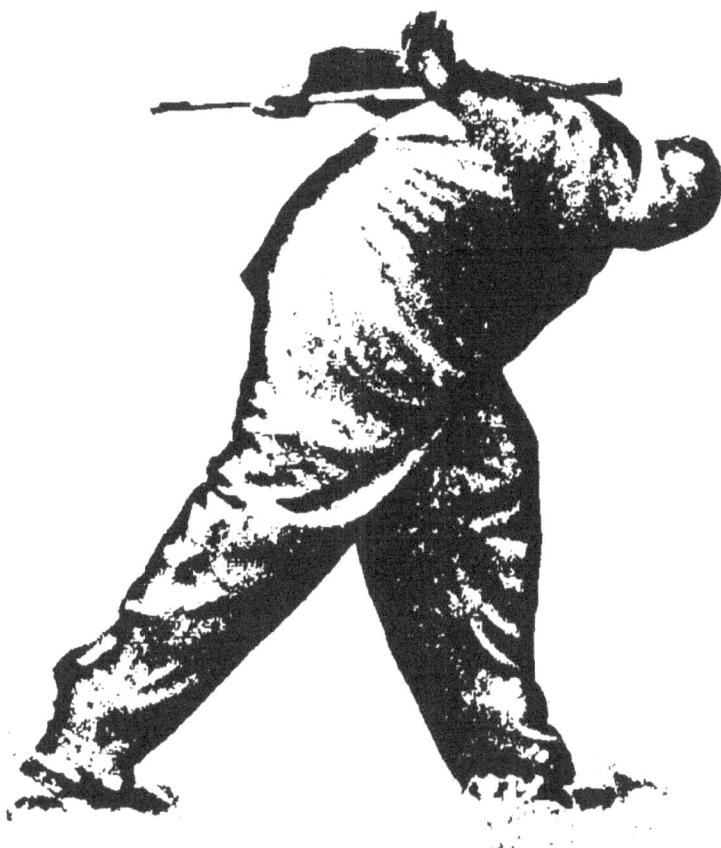

R.                                    L.

# A-ROM #18(A.) Crane spreads his right wing open.
## (Exa. 17)

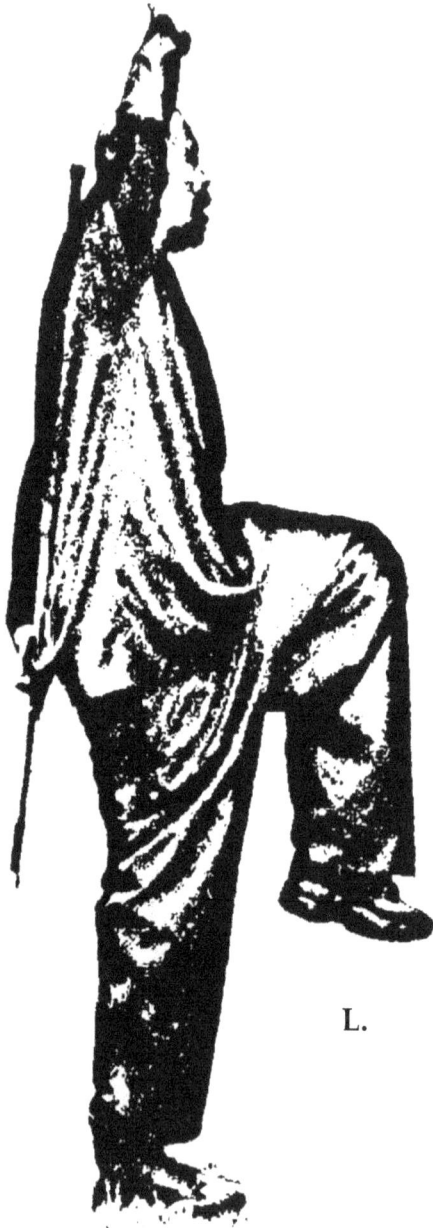

L.

R.

# A-ROM #18(B.) Crane spreads his right wing open.
## (Exa. 18)

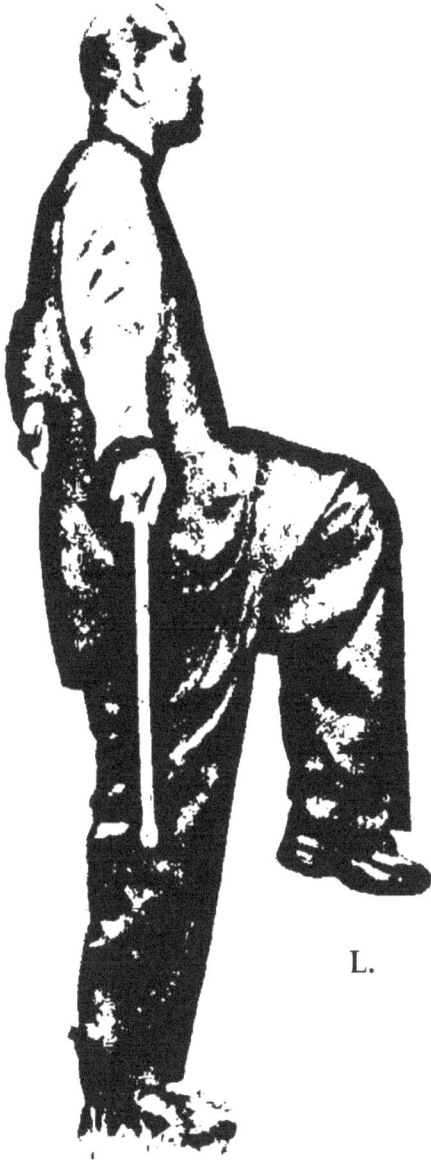

L.

R.

# A-ROM #19 Angry bird flaps his wings.
## (Exa. 19)

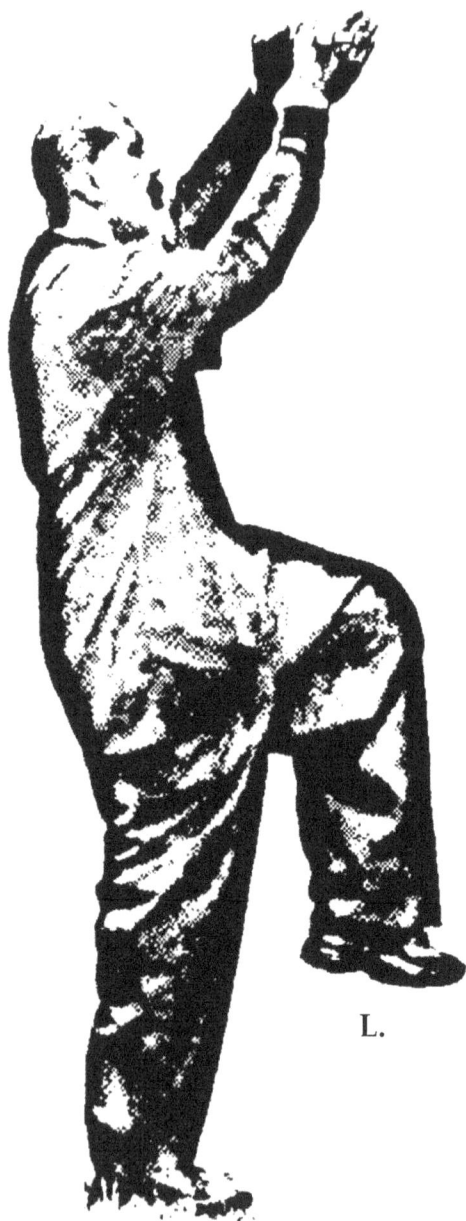

L.

R.

## (Exa. 20)

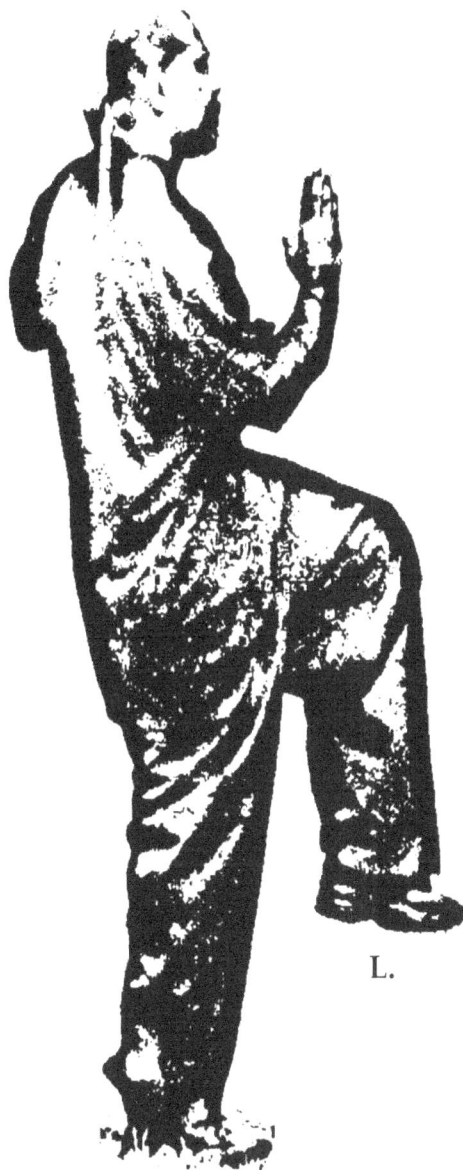

L.

R.

# The Ready Position pt. IV

Ἄλφα καὶ Ὠμέγα-(ἀρχή, & τὸ τέλος)

   In our last look at, *"The Ready Position,"* you will find that the body's weight distributes evenly on both legs. As you strive to find your centre, remember that the body is still in motion (*flux*). This is evident from the constant efforts to obtain balance (*poise*). Adding the **Staff**, **Spear**, or **Cane** to this equation will drive the body to seek its **Equilibrium,** or. (**equipoise**).

---

**Alpha & Omega** = Alfa y Omega (comienzo, fin &)

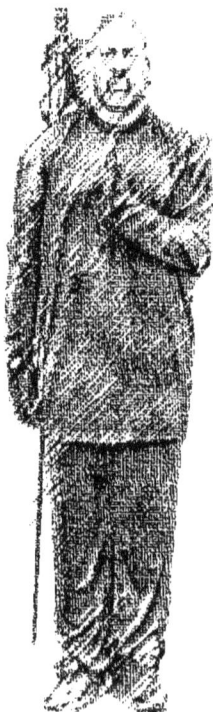

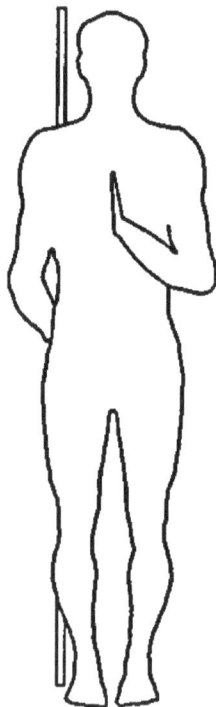

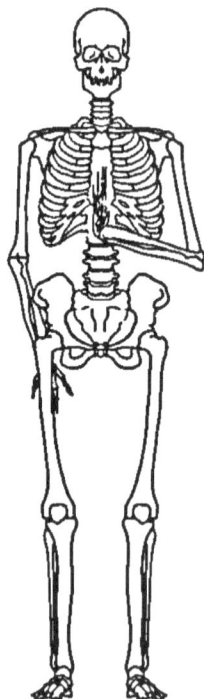

# Alpha & Omega, *a.k.a.* A & Ω
## *The Ready Position* - *(The Beginning & The End)*

A & Ω

科
技
Ω
开
始
科
技
结
束

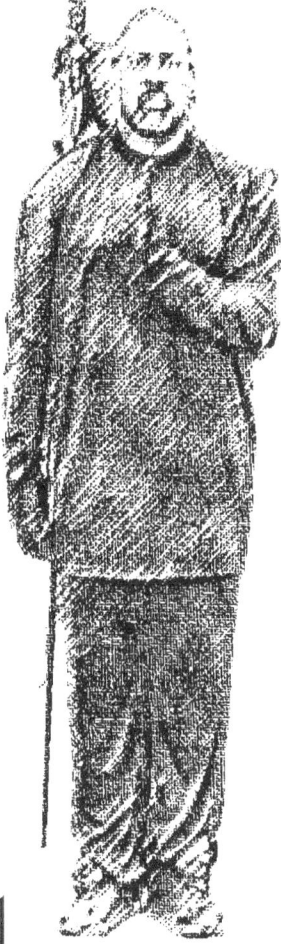

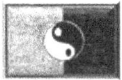

light    dark

r.       l.

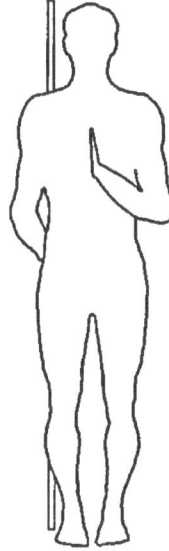

已
准
备
好
的
位
置
即

N

W        E

S

yang     yin
-------  -------
right    left

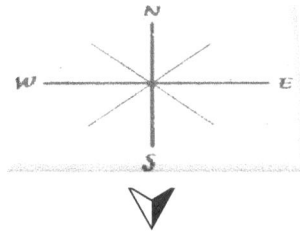

*Yin and Yang give way to one another,*
*in ways that their paths are forever, and infinite.*

# Chapter #4 Review

Walking Stick & Cane

Range of Motion a.k.a. ( ROME )

Adduction

Abduction

Flexion

Extension

Variance of Motion

Mechanics of Motion

Skeleton of The Human Body

Synovial Joints


**The Ready Position Pt. III** ( *Muscles & Parts of the Human Body* )


**Active Range Of Motion** ( A-ROM )


**The Ready Position Pt. IV** ( *Alpha & Omega* )

# Altered States

The mind does not change so much as we are led to believe. Within the process of our flow, we have knowledge of space, time, and reality. Because of this, we know also that, our thinking or thought process is the same accord, no matter what our present position is.

We are relaxed in our every aspect, maintaining the calmest collective. If possible, there is a relaxed and unattached feeling of sereneness, in our every action. Being hurried about any action is absent, thus eliminated. It is essential to be simplistic, in our methodical process.

As we assess,
we process.

我们评估我们处理

# Chapter 5.

## Mental & Physical Reconditioning

### The Crane Form **Part 4**
### Simplified Daily Exercise Routine

---

## Motor Set

To be motor set, robs the flow of its continuity, and spontaneity. You must entrain yourself to have Neuro-Muscular Conception. Be totally aware of the muscle, and its movement. This malfunction causes the spirit to find a resting place, an abode. The spirit that has a resting place is quick to anger. It becomes a mind and body that is motor set, in its own movement. You see, there is nothing more beautiful than the human body in motion, but of all the muscles in the human body, the mind is the most powerful.

# Wei Shen Do
## CH'ANG CHIEH CH'UAN
# &
# The Tao of Wu Wei

It is very important to understand, that the mind works in diverse ways. As the thought process unfolds, we are challenged to find answers to these events as they develop. If one is to advance, and find answers, you must be willing to *adapt, change, assimilate, transcend.* Knowing this, and executing it as mentioned earlier, is difficult to do. For anyone dealing with extreme change, he or she will no doubt encounter such obstacles. The individual that is willing to take the appropriate steps, is more likely to succeed. It is a matter of **completeness.** The fundamental principles are laid out before us, as with anything we do in life. It is our task to follow the path as it is laid out, or act upon it in a manner that will yield a positive effect. Any effort to indulge in negative thinking, or the like, will yield a mind that is destined to be motor set. By this I mean stagnate, in your efforts to advance, thus living a life that will be unfulfilling.

The first step is to analyze your illness, = (**opponent**). Careful considerations exist in this process. When viewing the actions of your illness, you must look past your own connotations, and view the disease for what it really is. You are being challenged to maintain control of your mind, body, and spirit. For this reason I view it as a battle between proponent, and opponent. **I.E.** (*Yang & Yin*) = (*good & evil*).

Looking at this in a closer analysis, you are fighting against the disease itself for control of your mind, body, and spirit. In any battle there is an opposition, or opposing side.

*The autoimmune disease itself is an affliction, that has attacked what was once a healthy body.*

## Illness = *opponent, etc.*

**YIN**

1. Aggressor
2. Assailant
3. Adversary
4. Antagonist

**NEGATIVE**

*Turn your chance hitting options of inabilities, into deliberate strikes of absolute capabilities...*

## Individual = *proponent, etc.*

**YANG**

1. Advocate
2. Exponent
3. Protagonist
4. Purest

**POSITIVE**

---

**ACTION** - (Wei - active) = *lively, vigorous, energetic.*

**NON** - (Wu - devoid) = *empty, barren, bereft, lacking.*

**PATH** - (Tao - direction) = *bearing, course, track, route.*

# Yin 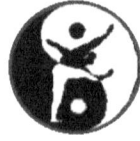 Yang

Dark                                                                Light

| Yielding | | Firmness |
| Deconstruction | | Constructive |
| Hard | | Soft |
| Insubstantial | | Substantial |
| Antagonist | | Protagonist |

## Opponent                          ## Proponent

Receptive                                                    Creative

Adversary                                                    Allies

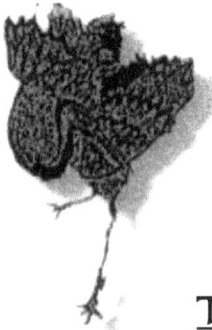

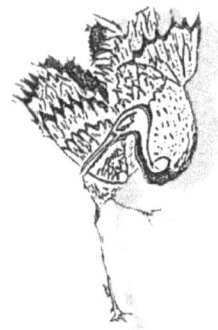

*6 feet, or 72 in.*
## The Basic Staff

Perception in a particular skill can improve by developing a training program that will emphasize specific traits of agility, and neuromuscular conditioning that enhance the relative skill or activity unconsciously.

# The following are techniques that I use, to help fight the negative effects of my illness.

---

1. Improve concentration and attention span.
2. Deal with the negative emotions of:

   A. Anger
   B. Hate
   C. Greed
   D. Lust

3. The acquisition and perfection of new skills.
4. Reprogramming, and anticipation of performance.
5. Total and complete relaxation before, and during.
6. The overall development of rhythm and timing.
7. The assimilation of more rapid and fluid motion.
8. The association of more efficient performance.
9. Improve body, and balance control of the skill.
10. Accurate perception of **space, time, and reality**.

The skilled individual is one who can adapt, and control coordinated movement patterns without having to think them through. As you advance in skill, and ability, the assimilation of complicated, and simple movement patterns changes, from conscious control to unconscious reflexes.

## Authors Note

In the following **14pages**, differentiate between **Yin & Yang**. This process is most important, as it will guide you in the tactics of determining the path. **opponent vs. proponent = illness vs. individual**

# Commitment - kə'mitmənt

*Taking in every aspect,*
*as you analyze its methods,*
*there are no limits to your measure.*

*This is to say your mind is* **<u>untethered</u>**...

**#1** Having analyzed the measure of commitment in the opponent's methods, you can foresee when he will relinquish the committal of his methods.

**#2** Once the opponent has committed himself, he has relinquished the right to move in and out freely, without restrain.

**#3** If you can measure the amount of force the adversary has committed to his actions, he will relinquish the advantage, by over committing himself.

**#4** Having foiled the flow of the aggressor, his actions can no longer be committed; thus, he has become the subject of fatigue, and must relinquish. The aggressor has exhausted himself.

**Measuring is applied through assessment...**
Assess the illness, and determine what you must do to win.

# Fixation - fik'seijn

*There is no pre-set fixation to how you must measure.*
*Development of the course,*
*is controlled by the actions of your adversary.*

**1.** Seek out the substantial, allowing the chain of events to follow along its course.

---

**2.** Such measures rely on the skill you adopt, while in the act of being formless.

---

**3.** Any altercation is an evaluation of necessity.

---

A. **Vernal** = Spring = Spry
B. **Vantage** = Superior = Omni
C. **Vanguard** = Leading = Ahead

---

i. Is such momentum - **effective.**
ii. Is such momentum - **advanced.**
iii. Is such momentum - **considerable.**

# Execution - əksəˈkjuːjn

To devise a means of execution,
a feasible method must be, **executed.**

1. Being prepared     A. Preparation
2. Being strategic    B. Strategy
3. Being mobile       C. Maneuvering

# Equivalence - ikwivələns

To devise a means of equivalence,
a feasible method must be, **equalized.**

---

**Seize ≥** 1. Being equal to or greater than the adversary.
**Fight**

---

**Caution ≤** 2. Being weaker than or close to adequate.
**Careful**

---

**Escaping ≈** 3. Being injured or unable to maneuver.
**Flee**

# Structure - strʌktfə

It does not matter how structured your tactics are,
if you lack the ability to execute, you will lose the advantage.

1. Direct vs. Compound = Simplicity
2. Mental vs. Physical = Cognitive
3. Aggressive vs. Passive = Calmness

Water has no feasible structure until it is contained in some shaped form or fixed fashion. Your actions cannot be measured in such a way that, the opponent will construct a means of containing the unattainable. If we must strive to have no form and be formless, our action is that of water, which cannot give way to any shaped form or fixed fashion.

# Control - kən;trəul

If you can learn to control the muscles that you would normally use, and relax the ones not being used at that time, your actions will be more fluid. The muscles will remain at rest until needed. Any attempt to flex or contract the muscle beforehand will result in a loss of reaction time. This tensing of the muscles slows down the neuromuscular activity between the mind, and the body. Total freedom of the mind allows for all out relaxation. An awareness that is completely relaxed and free, will move the body to a place where the spirit has, no abode.

# Engaging - inˈgeidʒiŋ

Excessive training cannot overcome common sense...
Dispose of the adversary with expedient means...

### 1. Direct Motion
### 2. Simple Motion
### 3. Efficient Motion

**The advance is lost if you have no
knowledge of how, and why, you engage...**

Applying multiple advances is a matter of deduction. Carry out your intent swiftly and move on to the next objective. When you have doubt, there is a moment of pausing in your process. Measuring of time is Instantaneous.

### 1. Hesitation causes doubt...
### 2. Stagnation causes doubt...

---

Acting aggressively dilutes the intent.
Act with the unconscious of intentions.

Your illness is the ***negativity*** within you.
Turn **negative** energy into **positive** energy.
Your persona becomes the ***positivity*** within you.

# The Three Actions

If the action is possible, it is best
to win without ever having fought at all.

If the action is possible, it is best
to have only what you need, disregard all else.

If the action is possible, it is best
to have understanding of the unknown.

---

# The Five Possibilities

If possible, have the opposition
follow you in a way that is absolute.

If possible, choose your battles.
Lead, but do not follow.

If possible, know the path
and direction you partake. **Hard or Soft.**

If possible, your adaptation
should lead to a position of opportunity.

If possible, the chain of events,
is followed in the course it is given.

# The Explanation of Terms

*The following words, and definitions are listed in alphabetical order. You will find the terms, and explanations to be slightly different from what you have come to know. Adapt, Change, Assimilate, and Transcend them into your daily activity.*

<u>ANALYZE</u> - Analyze the opponent and make him give in such a way, that he has no focus on where his next move will be. Such actions give the opponent no other way of presenting himself.

<u>ANGER</u> - Use the opponent's emotional content to throw him off his guard. Anger him, as a way of measuring his intentions.

<u>APPROPRIATE</u> - Take the offensive, as an act of conditioning that will not allow the opponent the will to advance. Do what is necessary to insure your resolution.

<u>ASSESSMENT</u> - Take advantage of the opponent at every angle. Form a means of entrapment, to seize him into your plight. Whatever he has, available to him should be yours. Victory is easy for those of us who plan for it, while defeat, is easy for those of us, who do not plan to be victorious.

<u>CHANGE</u> - You must change the course of action taken by the opponent in such a way, that he will find himself prohibited. Lead him into feeling unsure of his every action.

**COMPLETE** - It is important to know that winning or even being successful must first incorporate a plan of completeness. How can you succeed, if you have no forethought to your actions?

**CONCENTRATION** - When you are focused and have direction, you are united. When the opponents divided and has no purpose, you will out think him or outnumber him.

**CONDITIONS** - This is defined as the amount of effort, you apply to every action. Be it fast or slow, hard or soft, light or heavy, but is also governed by the methods of your opponent.

**CONSTANT** - As there is a constant in the universe, like wise your actions are like water, flowing, and changing its shape and form.

**DECEPTION** - For the purest, it is a matter of execution. Appearing to be something, you are not, as a means of being withdrawn. To engage when you are appearing to be supple is evasive.

**DEPLETION** - You must deplete your opponent's action in such a way, that he has nothing left to use at his disposal. He will exhaust every option, and be defeated.

**DESPERATION** - The action is as stated, when the opponent has depleted himself, he will do whatever he has to, as a desperate act of survival.

**DESTRUCTION** - For the individual that is skillful, he knows that destroying his opponent will bring about his destruction. To cut him off at every turn, without pause is strategic.

**DISTANCE** - The methods you employ must incorporate an action that is based on illusion. Distance is accomplished by drawing the unwanted guard. The aggressor is fooled by immeasurable acts.

**DISTRACTION** - With the intent to find out the lengths of which your opponent will go, you must alter his attention span to deduce his actions.

**DRAWING** - When the opponent has been given the illusion that he has won, he has actually been fooled, by the emotions of greed and lust. One cannot prosper by ill intent to the opponent. Any victory that is won by force is a victory that is won by ill intent, which is considered negative.

**EFFICIENT** - The best laid plan is one that is simple and direct, where there is no way in which to deduce the actions. These and other such actions are unexpected motions.

**EMPTINESS** - You are ready and not bothered, with the prospect of gaining an advantage over your opponent's engagement of you.

**ENDLESS** - It would appear that your actions know no boundaries. You have managed to release your very essence upon your opponent.

**ENDURANCE** - The aggressor knows that to over extend or exhaust the limits while engaging, will bring about insufficient motions. You should know this as well. For the purest, it is a matter of being spontaneous. To win, you must be direct, and unattainable.

**FORCE** - The force that you apply is likened, to that of water rushing down a mountain. The limits of such actions can be limitless.

**FORM** - The form that you choose is one that follows the methods of your opponent's actions. You do not reveal yourself until he does.

**FULLNESS** - To arrive first, is to distinguish between what is necessary, and what is inaccurate. Stationary but not stagnant is the key.

**HUMBLE** - As you give the appearance of being defeated, you imply your shame of losing. This causes the opponent to be self-indulged by his greed. Attack the unknowing, with unexpected humility.

**INFINITY** - To be without any plausible means of ever ending, you have reached a state of which is almost indefinable.

**INFLUENCE** - By altering the opponent in such a way, you invoke him into your void. Making your opponent feel inane gives birth to your fulfillment.

**LENGTH** - In terms of distance, we mean to say direction. How far will you go to attain your goal? What actions will you take, to finalize the intent? Being near but being far and unreachable. (Vice versa).

**LOCATION** - You must centralize to a specific space, time, and reality, where your actions are those of the purest. Reaching but not over extending to localize. The Purest establishes his diversion, which is his ability to be centered, by applying division.

**MANIPULATE** - There is a confusion of the opponent's perception of what is and what you led him not to believe. When given the unexpected, he is lost in a state of disarrayed motions.

**METHODS** - This is the course of action you will use, be it mental or physical. The result, involves precepts of which we use to accomplish the objective. To gain an advantage over your foe, methodical efforts must prevail, or the advantage is lost.

**OPPOSITION** - As a standard rule. never face the aggressor whose field of motion is cut off, in a way that he cannot retreat. This is to say give him enough room to defeat himself.

**PERSISTENCE** - Engage the opponent, but do not seek reward in being excessive. The application is the amount needed to dispel the initiator, in the most practical or pragmatic of ways.

**PREPARATION** - We must organize ourselves in such a way, to be invincible against every aspect. Your main concern should focus on being ready, for what is about to take place. In the act of knowing ourselves, we give rise to the formation of intrinsic knowledge of ourselves.

**SPACE** - In the process of measuring, you should be aware of the area, and the amount of effort it takes to maneuver from one space to another. Survey as a whole and not as a segregated piece.

**STRATEGIC** - To have a flawless victory, you must undergo a series of precognitive acts, which overwhelm the opponent without having used any means of physical force.

**STRENGTH** - When the opponent is obviously stronger than you are, it is wise to avoid his oppositions. Engage him in an unorthodox manner.

**SUPERIORITY** - For the purest, it is a matter of knowing when to advance, and when to retreat. Question him, when he is advancing; answer him, as he is retreating.

**SWIFTNESS** - Your actions are like those of the wind, moving in the most expedient of means, you execute without any haste. Be it fast or slow, hard or soft the motions are light and supple. The application of any motion is performed to the maximum, by the means of not being seen, felt or even heard.

**UNEXPECTED** - To be spontaneous in execution is the act of penetration. You have acquired a stroke that is un-easily detected until felt. The opponent could not see, feel, or hear your intent.

<u>UNFAILING</u> - The Purest is victorious because he manages to approach each confrontation, with methods of which the opponent cannot seem to alter or adapt.

<u>UNORTHODOX</u> - By the process of elimination, The proponent has expanded his limits, and learned to exceed them; by being in a continual flux of residual and transitional motion.

<u>USAGE</u> - When you engage the opposition in such a way as to cause him to act upon himself, your own action will appear to be stronger, than those of your adversary. Yin and Yang give way to one another by conjoining, in a way that their paths are forever and infinite.

<u>VICTORY</u> - While in the chain of events, it is important to remember the overall goal. To be absolute, without being self-absorbed.

<u>VULNERABLE</u> - Having a form that is yielding at an improper time, gives the opposition the ascension he so desperately wants. We must evaluate our methods as a form, and function of necessity. Applying the proper form and function at the proper time, gives rise to an unyielding force that is invulnerable.

# Chapter #5 Review

Wei Shen Do  &  The Tao of Wu Wei

Yin & Yang

Commitment -

Fixation -

Execution -

Equivalence -

Structure -

Control -

Engaging -

---

The Three Actions


The Five Possibilities


The Explanation of Terms

# The Purest

When we push the limits to exceed them, we do so not to exhaust them totally without residual.

When you administer the aforementioned, its success is out of strategy, not out of ordinary luck.

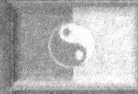

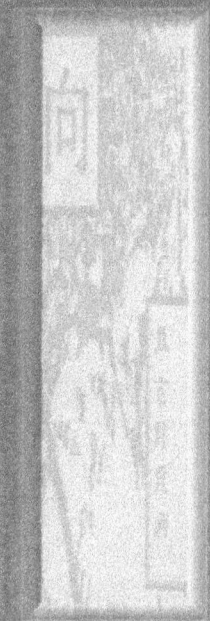

# Chapter 6.

## Physical Fitness
## &
## Training Methods

### The Crane Form <u>Part 5</u>
### Simplified Daily Exercise Routine

---

# To Flow

To Flow involves the precept of creation,

while at the same time decreasing negative actions.

Therefore our expansion,

would imply that we have increased our flow,

with daily decrease...

# Physical Activity

There are quite a few books on the subject of fitness, but this one has been written for those who suffer from limited movement, and range of motion issues. In this last chapter we will cover the benefits of warming up, and cooling down. We will also discuss physical fitness, training methods, and efficiency in execution. Fitness is driven by many factors. Such as genetic structure, and environmental elements that involve stress, nutrition, rest, and exercise. When considering the redevelopment of an individual after dealing with an injury, or recovering from a serious illness, you must look at or examine three distinct areas.

A. **Physique** = **build or structure** - *bone structure, fat, etc.*
B. **Organic** = **carbon-based** - *heart, lungs, kidney, etc.*
C. **Muscular** = **brawny** - *skeletal, muscular movement, etc.*

**Flexibility -** *Suppleness of the body as it advances in range of motion. Flowing and natural.*

**Strength -** *The amount of flexibility, speed, and endurance any muscle or its parts has in a combination of the latter.*

**Speed -** *Expand and contract a muscle through its range of motion without causing further injury.*

**Endurance -** *The amount of stress a muscle can endure before it reaches its maximum level.*

# Muscular Endurance

Power is the product of strength, and speed. As power is increased and attained, this will no doubt bring about the improvement of strength and speed. Muscle training increases muscle strength and speed of movement. Muscular endurance is a vital component of motion economy, and simplicity. Any amount of gain in the muscle, and its endurance can be increased through high repetitions and relative low resistance. All this and more must be considered when dealing with any disease that inhibits muscular development.

> **A.** *Most individuals fail to realize that a substantial amount of power must be repeated a number of times throughout each exercise.*

> **B.** *With a high level of endurance, the quality of the power released is maintained, thus the individual is still fresh at the time of execution.*

> **C.** *Endurance training should include several different systems of training. This is true in every aspect of development. Be it variety or physiological, anyone can benefit from it.*

**Cardiovascular Endurance -** *the ability of the body as a whole to sustain optimal performance of a particular skill for a prolonged length of time.*

**Endurance -** *the ability of an individual to sustain optimal performance, with the absence of fatigue or exhaustion while performing a specific skill, maneuver, or technique.*

**Local Endurance -** *the execution of work done by a relative muscle or exact group of muscles for an extended amount of time, of which fatigue is segregated to that particular group.*

# ʄlexibility

Flexibility is a very important part of fitness, but as with other elements of physical fitness it's importance is comparative. For example, the flexibility of one individual may differ from another. In general, improved flexibility enhances performance. Because of this, it can be viewed as an infinite medium that ranges from a few minutes of stretching, to a full thirty minutes. Flexibility is best achieved through stretching exercises, which are broken down into four categories:

**A.** *Static*
**B.** *Passive*
**C.** *Ballistic*
**D.** *Contracting - Relaxing*

Of these four, static is the safest. Static stretching incorporates slow gentle movements where the body uses its own weight to stretch specific muscles. For this sole purpose, static stretching is our primary concern, because it can reduce the chance of physical injury.

**A proper warm up may include any of the following.**

**A.** *Walking*
**B.** *Meditation*
**C.** *Stretching*
**D.** *Breathing*

**A proper warm up may also do any of the following.**

**A.** *Prepare the body for exercise.*
**B.** *Help prevent injury - reduce muscular soreness.*
**C.** *Increase blood flow - muscular temperature.*
**D.** *Prepare the individual mentally for activity.*

Learning to relax can be beneficial to stretching, and achieving flexibility. As a rule of thumb it is advised that you attempt to stimulate circulation first. Executing with fluid motion, start out with short movements, and work up to longer ranges of motion. Remember exercises can be performed in three primary positions. Standing, sitting, or lying down. Also remember to do these three things in conjunction.

**A.** *Breath*
**B.** *Concentrate*
**C.** *Focus*

If one is determined to achieve a sufficient range of motion, he or she must first develop flexibility through exercise. This is followed by strength building exercises that lead to speed, and endurance. A muscle should be flexible enough to allow for full range of motion. If you have flexibility, and strength, you have speed, and endurance.

**The Crane Form** is a perfect example of static exercise. Another aspect to static stretching is that you are in a fixed position for a specific amount of time. Such exercises as The Crane Form, can be done with or without the aid of a partner, and done with or without a staff or cane. Learn the basic form, and then build upon its principle segments.

**A proper cool down may involve, or do any of the following.**

**A.** *Continue Activity at a lower intensity.*
**B.** *Slow the heart rate down to 100 beats a minute.*
**C.** *Allows breathing and heart rate to return to normal.*
**D.** *Minimize soreness and stiffness for the next day.*
**E.** *Cool down under normal conditions of 4 to 6 min….*

# The Warm Up

Warm-up principles are vital to physical health. The main purpose of warming up is to increase your heart rate slightly. This has two benefits:

**A.** *Raise your body temperature.*

**B.** *Increases the blood (oxygen) flow to your muscles, to prepare the body for vigorous movement.*

Your muscles and tendons are more receptive to stretching after a light warm-up raises your internal body temperature. This will help you to increase the range of motion in your joints, and help you to avoid further injuries. Focus your warm up on large muscle groups, then smaller ones.

The substantial increase in blood flow to the skeletal muscles make them supple, and more adaptable to stretching. With an increase in blood flow the muscles consistently increase the amount of oxygen and other nutrients. The warm-up also jump starts the neuromuscular system between the nervous system, and various muscle groups. A light warm up generally last from eight to ten minutes. Skeletal muscles and their groups are more susceptible to strain, and tearing if the muscles are aggressively stretched without a warm up.

*The warm-up should be intense enough to increase your body temperature, but not strenuous enough to cause fatigue.*

# The Cool Down

**A.** *Stopping suddenly can cause light - headedness.*

**B.** *The cool down serves three purposes:*

    **1.** *It reduces your pulse.*
    **2.** *It returns the blood to your heart.*
    **3.** *Reduce the amount of **Lactic Acid**.*
      *A chemical result of muscular fatigue.*

**C.** *If you stop suddenly, the blood will settle in your legs instead of returning to your heart.*

**D.** *It takes your body about 3 minutes to stop pumping extra blood to your muscles. A safe cool down is about 3 minutes, give or take 4 - 5 minutes.*

As of today there is no tangible indication, that cooling down reduces what is known as ***delayed onset muscle soreness (DOMS)***. This condition frequently occurs in muscles that have been exposed to a vigorous workout, with the commencement of muscle discomfort un-present for 24 to 48 hours. As a general rule, a simple and effective means of cooling down is to continue to exercise at a low intensity level for 8 to 10 minutes. As stated in the latter, the evidence is inconclusive, as to whether or not cooling down will in fact deter the onset of **DOMS**, but the amount of residual gain in suppleness is very evident.

# The Twelve Daily Exercises

*These 12 exercises should be performed on a daily basis.*

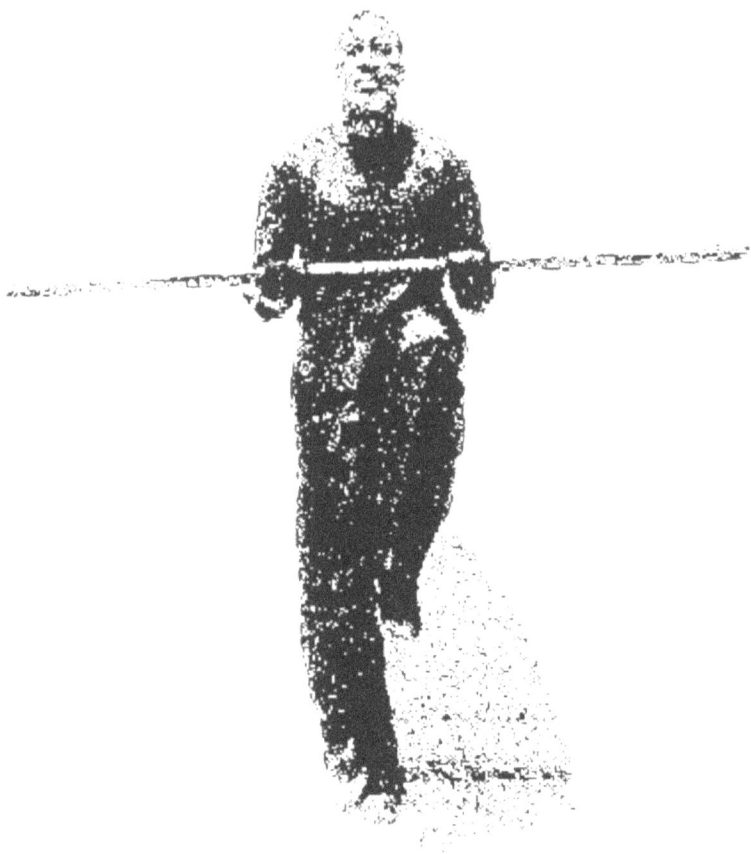

After my last ER visit I immediately started training my mind, body, and spirit all over again. I picked my brain trying to put together the intrinsic pieces of the puzzle. Within the months that followed I established what is now **The Twelve Daily Exercises**. Each exercise was created from some of the basic exercises, and fitness routines that have been around for over thousands of years. Each one is unique because it can be altered to fit people from all walks of life. From young or old, to disabled & incapacitated.

# Hand Placements & Positions

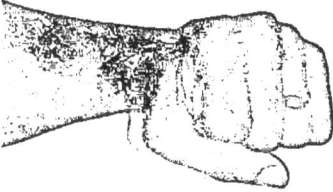

**OVERHAND GRIP**

*The thumb is down.*

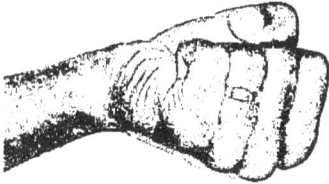

**UNDERHAND GRIP**

*The thumb is up.*

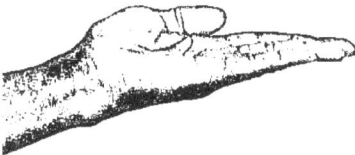

**SUPINATION**

*The palm facing upward.*

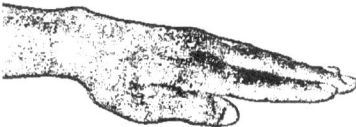

**PRONATION**

*The palm facing downward.*

*Please refer back to page 82 of this text for a precise definition of hand placements, and positioning's.*

# Exercise 1. Marching In Place

**1.**

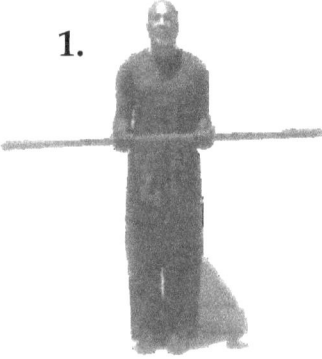

r. l.

**2.**

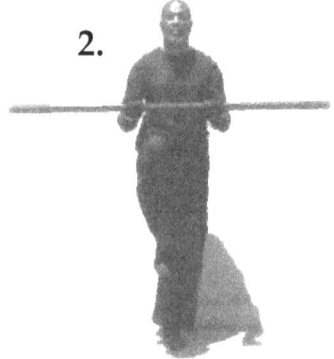

r. l.

Start the exercise with both feet planted firmly to the ground. Your hands are placed in a underhand position holding the staff a shoulders length apart in the centre. On the count of two you raise your right foot. On the count of three you raise your left foot, and lower your right foot. On the count of four you return back to the starting position with both feet on the ground. Repeat this exercise until you become tired. Concentrate on building up speed, and endurance.

**3.**

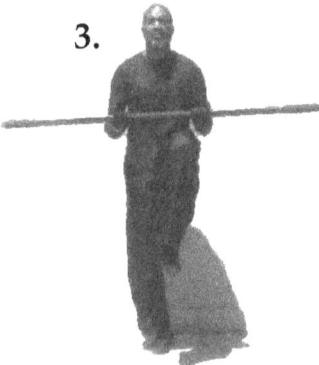

r. l.

**4.**

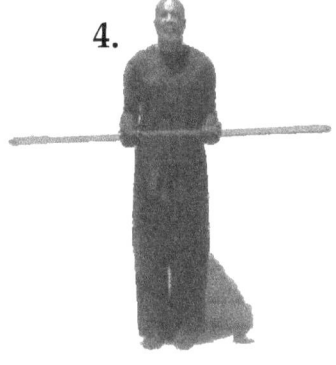

r. l.

# Exercise 2. Biceps Curl

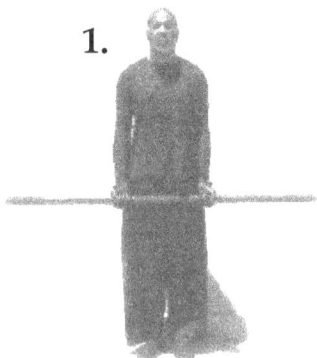

1.

r. l.

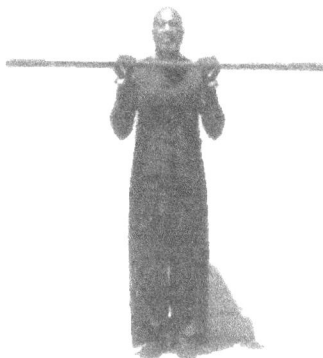

2.

r. l.

Hold the staff in the center with a underhand grip. On the count of one both hand are a shoulders length apart, with both arms extended and hanging down. Raise the staff to your neck on the count of two, bending at the elbows. While in the same position bring both hands above your head to exercise three. From position one you bring both hands behind your neck to position two.

# Exercise 3. Triceps Curl

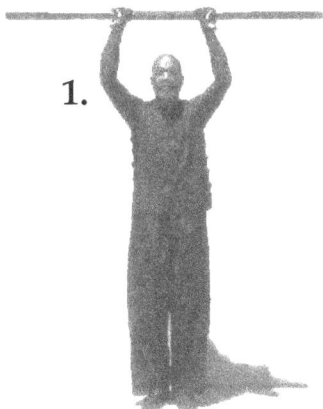

1.

r. l.

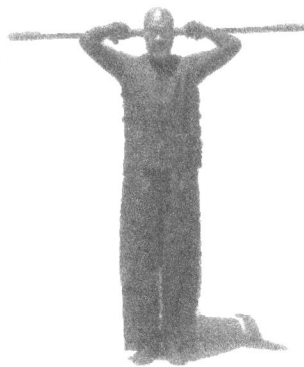

2.

r. l.

# Exercise 4. Figure 8 Right Hand

1.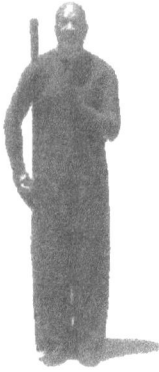

r. l.

2.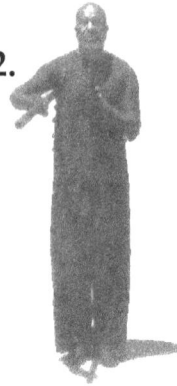

r. l.

Starting in The Ready Position, the right arm brings the staff horizontal to the ground to position two.  From position three you turn the staff vertical to a pronated position, and proceed to position four turning the staff once again to a horizontal position.  With the hand in an overhand grip (pronated) from position four, you proceed to position five.

3.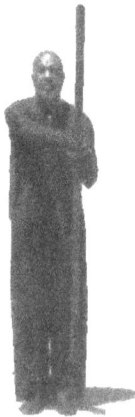

r. l.

4.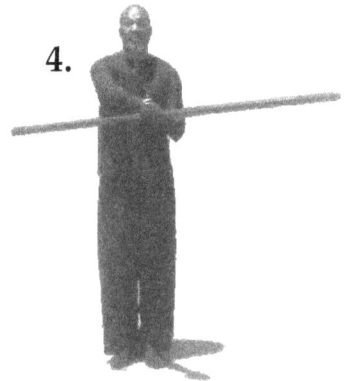

r. l.

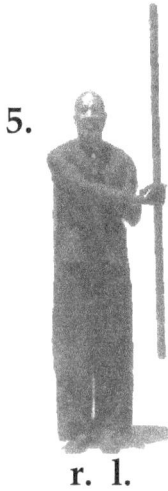

5. r. l.

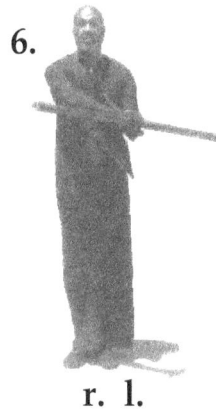

6. r. l.

Starting from position five in a supinated grip from the left the staff is held vertically. In position six rotate the staff until it is horizontal. As you move the staff to the right your hand pronates into position seven. You end with your hand holding the staff vertically in front of the body in position eight. From here you can tuck the staff back behind your right shoulder.

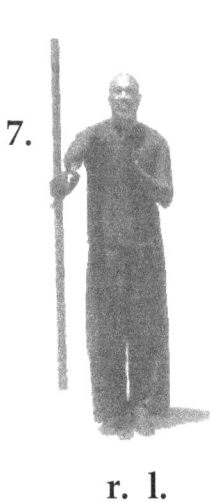

7. r. l.

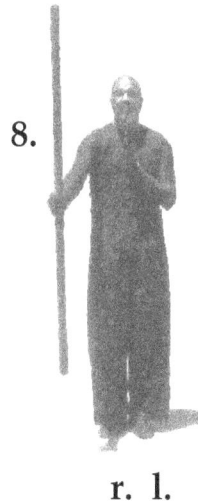

8. r. l.

# Exercise 5. Figure 8 Left Hand

1.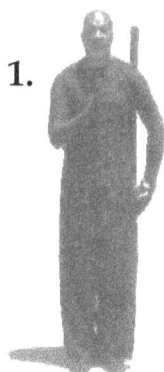

2.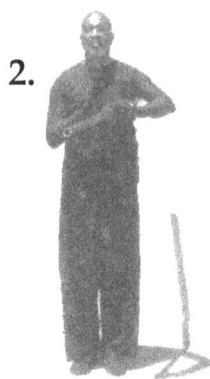

r. l.                                    r. l.

Starting in The Ready Position, the left arm brings the staff horizontal to the ground to position two. From position three you turn the staff vertical to a pronated position, and proceed to position four turning the staff once again to a horizontal position. With the hand in an overhand grip (pronated) from position four, you proceed to position five.

3.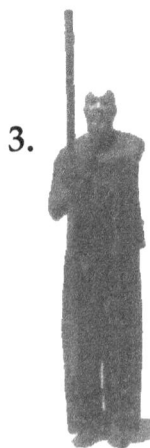

4.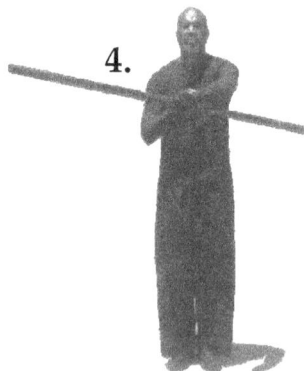

r. l.                                    r. l.

5.

r. l.

6.

r. l.

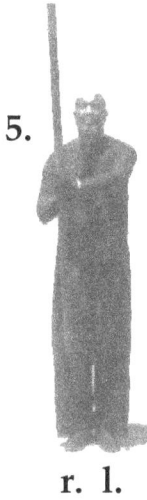

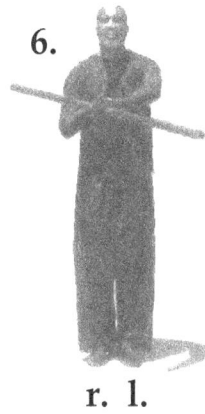

Starting from position five in a supinated grip from the right the staff is held vertically. In position six rotate the staff until it is horizontal. As you move the staff to the left your hand pronates into position seven. You end holding the staff vertically in front of the body in position eight. From here you can tuck the staff back behind your left shoulder.

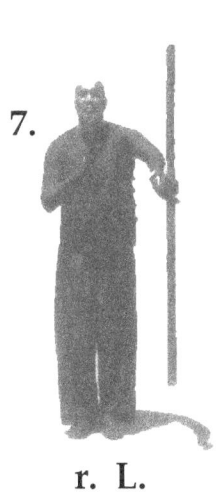

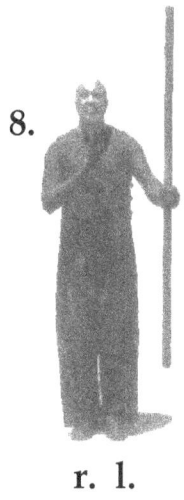

7.

r. L.

8.

r. l.

# Exercise 6. Left Hand Twirl

**1.**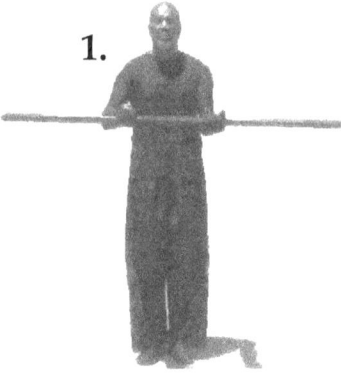

**2.**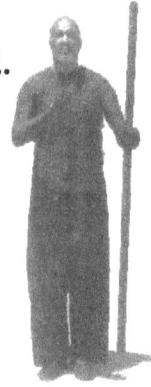

r. l.                                    r. l.

Starting from position one with both hands in a underhand grip. Release the pole out of your right hand and let it drop. In position two as the pole drops, let it hang as you hold it vertically in front of your body, with the left hand. Your right hand comes to a proximal position in front of your chest. From position three turn the pole up to the left, and bring it to a horizontal position. Position four ends with your left hand turning the staff up to a vertical position, as your right hand grabs the staff in the middle.

**3.**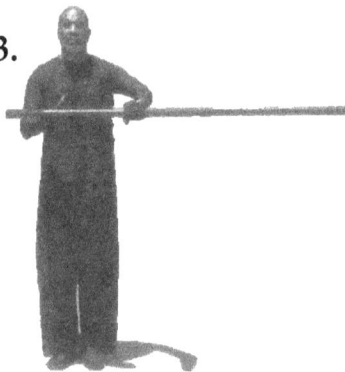

**4.**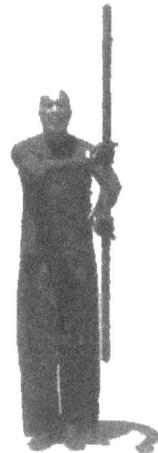

r. l.                                    r. l.

# Exercise 7. Right Hand Twirl

**1.**

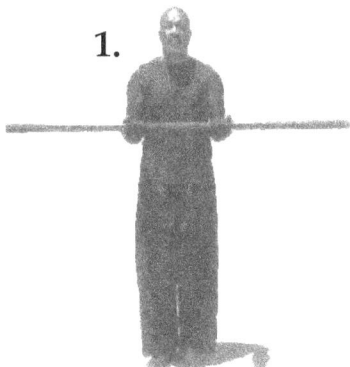

r. l.

**2.**

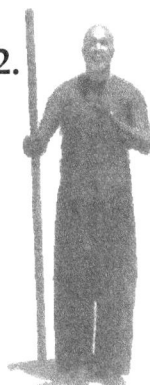

r. l.

Starting from position one with both hands in a underhand grip. Release the pole out of your left hand and let it drop. In position two as the pole drops, let it hang as you hold it vertically in front of your body, with the right hand. Your left hand comes to a proximal position in front of your chest. From position three turn the pole up to the left, and bring it to a horizontal position. Position four ends with your right hand turning the staff up to a vertical position, as your left hand grabs the staff in the middle.

**3.**

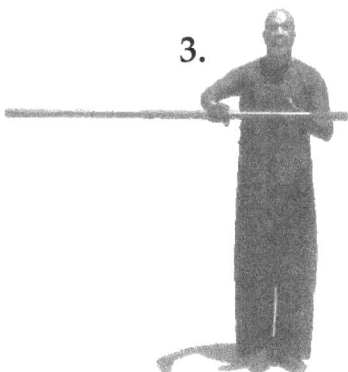

r. l.

**4.**

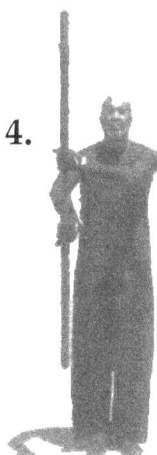

r. l.

# Exercise 8. Over Hand Swing Right

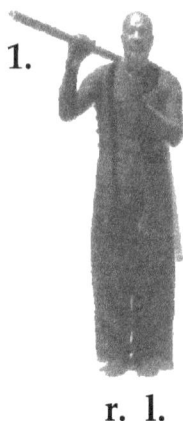

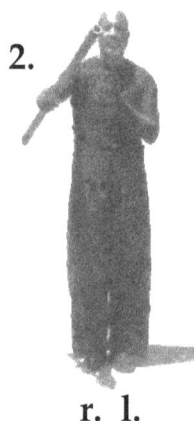

**1.**

r. l.

**2.**

r. l.

Starting from position one your right hand holds the staff horizontally over your right shoulder. In position two the staff comes over the shoulder past your head, and is pointing in front of your body horizontally. From position three you bring the staff down to a vertical position, with the right hand pronated. The last movement is position four, as the staff rest behind your right shoulder in The Ready Position.

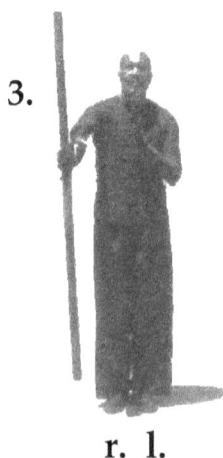

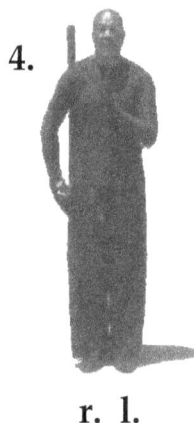

**3.**

r. l.

**4.**

r. l.

# Exercise 9. Over Hand Swing Left

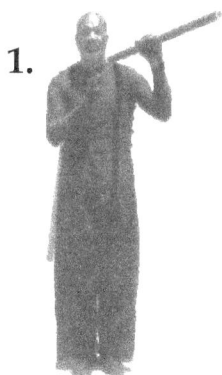

**1.**

r. l.

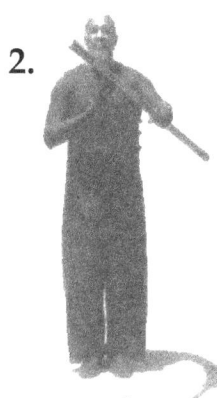

**2.**

r. l.

Starting from position one your left hand holds the staff horizontally over your left shoulder. In position two the staff comes over the shoulder past your head, and is pointing in front of your body horizontally. From position three you bring the staff down to a vertical position, with the left hand pronated. The last movement is position four, as the staff rest behind your left shoulder in The Ready Position.

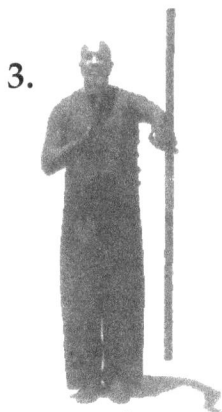

**3.**

r. l.

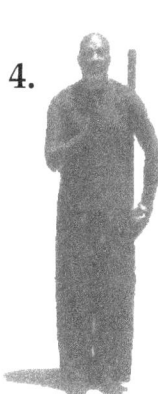

**4.**

r. l.

# Exercise 10. Mid-Section Twist

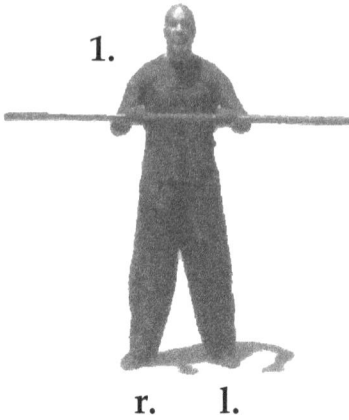

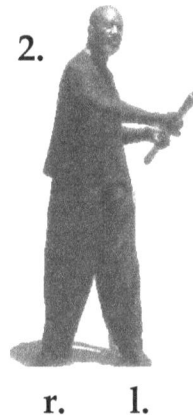

1.

2.

r.    l.          r.    l.

In position one hold the pole in the center with both hands placed in an overhand grip. Your feet are placed firmly on the ground a shoulders length apart, with the knees slightly bent. From here you proceed to position two, and turn your upper body slowly to the left. In position three you advance and turn to the right from position two. You end the exercise in position four as you turn your upper body back to the left facing forward. Repeat this exercise until you are tired.

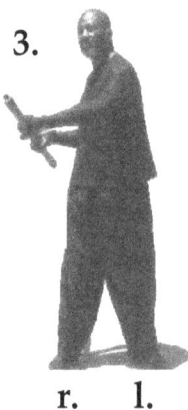

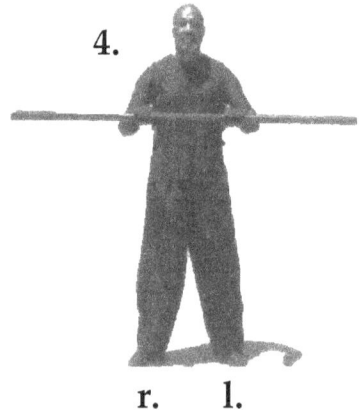

3.

4.

r.    l.          r.    l.

# Exercise 11. Ambidextrous Jab

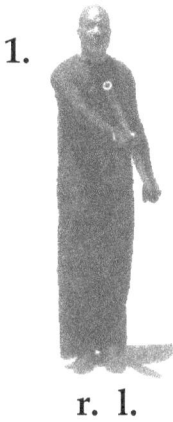

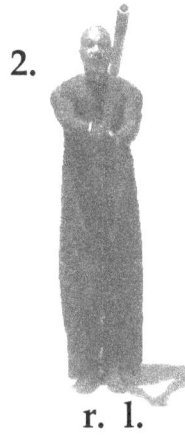

1.

r. l.

2.

r. l.

From position one hold the pole to the left of your body. Your left hand is held at the end, while your right hand grasp the centre. In position two you slide the pole through your right hand until your hands meet. As you release your grip in the right hand in position three, slide the pole back down with your right hand holding it to the right of your body. In position four slide the pole through your left hand until both hands meet. You end back where you started in position one.

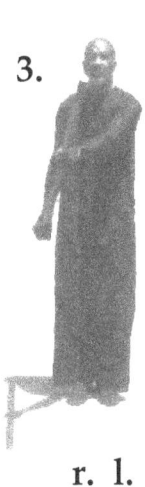

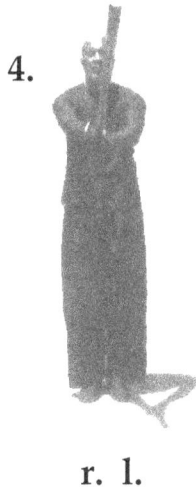

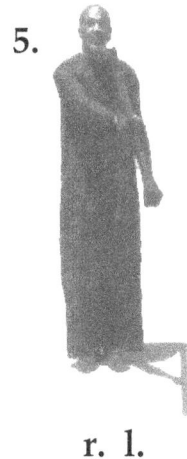

3.

r. l.

4.

r. l.

5.

r. l.

# Exercise 12. Left & Right Sweep

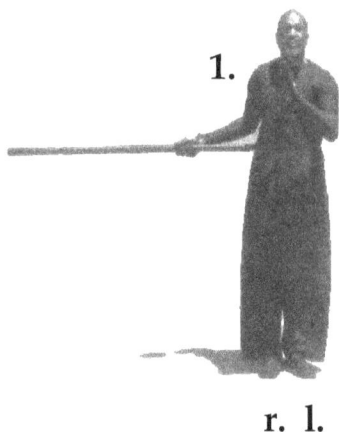

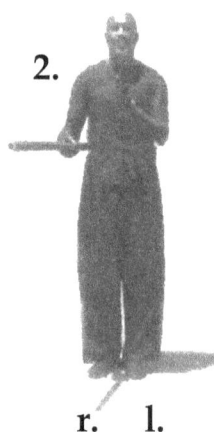

1.

r. l.

2.

r.    l.

Starting from the right in position one, you hold the staff out and away from your body horizontally. The left hand is held in front of the chest. As you bring the staff around horizontally, point it in front of your body to position two.  In position three swing the staff up and around until it is above your head, horizontal to the floor. Your left hand comes up and grabs the staff above your head. Both hands are crossed one in front of the other.  Releasing your grip in the right hand, you

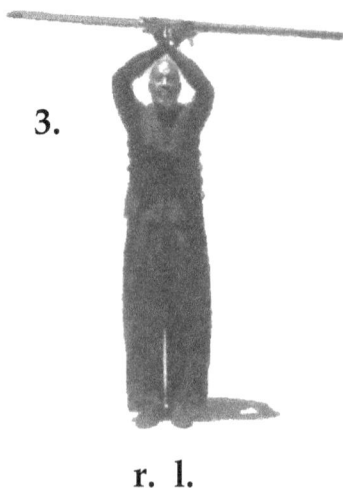

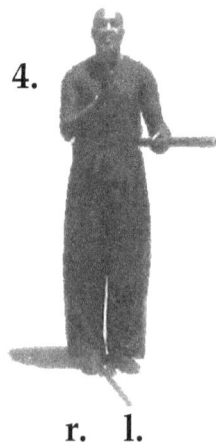

3.

r. l.

4.

r.    l.

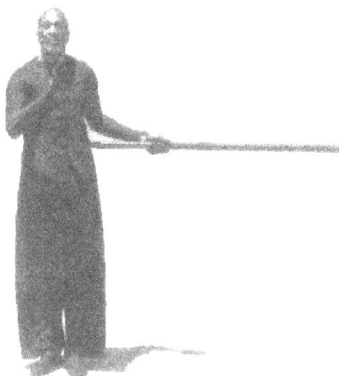

5.

r. l.

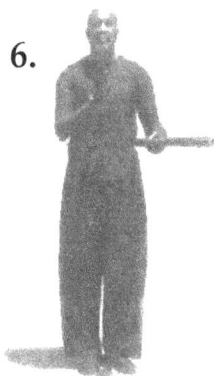

6.

r.    l.

grab the staff in your left hand, dropping your right hand down to your chest in position four. Position five is the reverse action, as you swing the staff out and away from your body to the left. Now in position six you bring the staff in front of your body, and continue to swing it up and around ending above your head in position seven. With both hands above your head you release your grip in the left hand, and grab the staff with your right. Ending in position eight the staff is now in front of your body in the right hand. Your left hand drops back down.

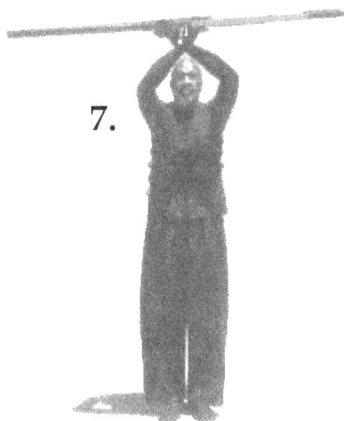

7.

r. l.

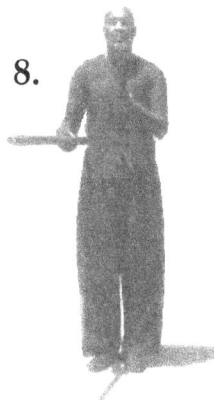

8.

r.    l.

# Bonus Exercise 13. Deep Knee Bends

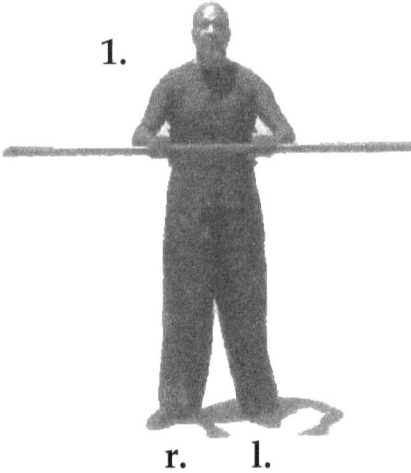

In this bonus exercise you can add it to your Twelve Daily Exercises as a personal goal to reach. Start out with both hands held out in front of you. Your hands are spread a shoulders width apart, in an overhand position. Both feet are placed firmly on the ground a shoulders width apart, with the knees slightly bent.

*Paying close attention to your balance, you slowly drop down to position two, bending your knees.*

Remember to keep your hands out in front of you to help maintain balance. Your feet should stay planted firmly to the ground, as you open up your legs. Hold for five seconds and return back to position one. Rise up slowly and repeat again.

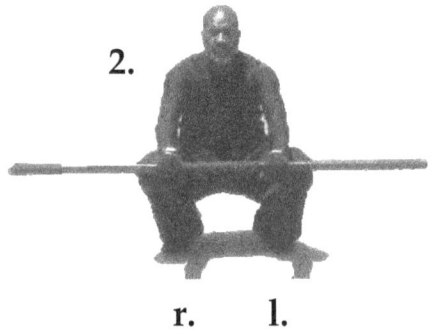

# Stretching

Stretching is one of the most neglected aspects of any exercise routine. This is due to the lack of knowledge that most people have about physical fitness.

## Methods to Follow

**A.** *Stretch the muscle until you can feel a pulling sensation in the middle.*

**B.** *Hold the stretch for 20 - 30 seconds.*

**C.** *If the pulling sensation ceases before the stretch is depleted, inhale, and re-exhale until you can feel it again. Relax the muscle, and repeat to advance further into the expansion.*

**D.** *All of the exercises shown are for numerous reasons. Stretching, flexibility, endurance, strength, mental, and physical relaxation.*

**E.** *After a few minutes as you begin to breathe easier, stretch while your muscles are still warm. This will aid in the elongation process of the muscles during the stretching segment.*

**F.** *Remember to Inhale as you move into your stretching position. As you exhale relax. Exhaling allows you to lengthen the connective tissues, which increases the effect of the stretch.*

**G.** *Stretching before and after any exercise segment, can help reduce muscle cramping, muscle soreness, and early morning stiffness. Stretching can also reduce further injury, and help relieve tension & stress.*

# Standing & Sitting Drill

A great exercise for people with limited movement.
*Exceptional for people who have trouble sitting for long periods of time.*

**1.**

**2.**

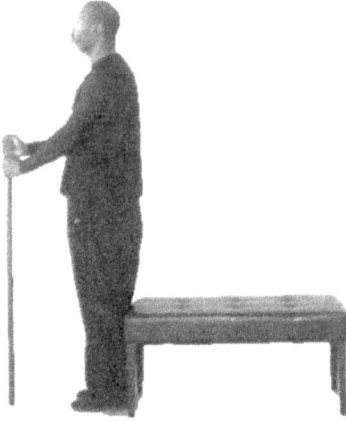

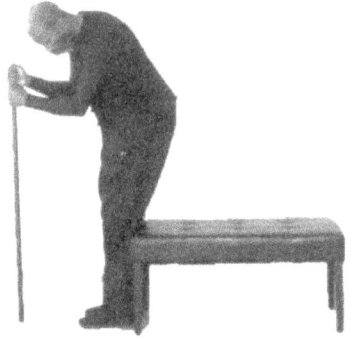

**5.**

**6.**

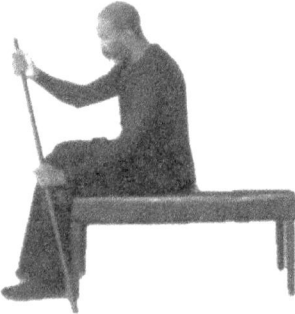

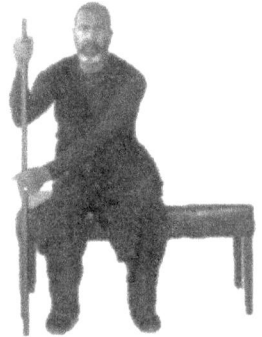

The following stretching routine can be performed in its entirety, or broken down to fit your needs. The routine consist of three short segments. Each one can be modified for any condition.

**3.**

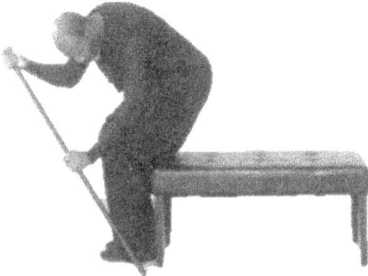

**4.**

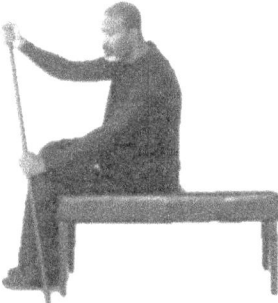

**7.**

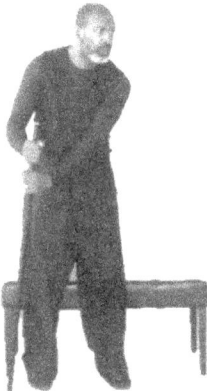

**8.**

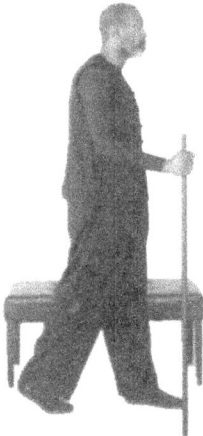

## Right Hamstring & Lower Back One

**1.**

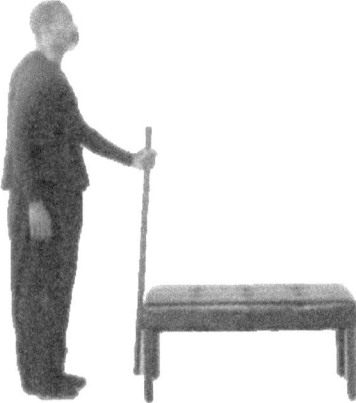

**2.**

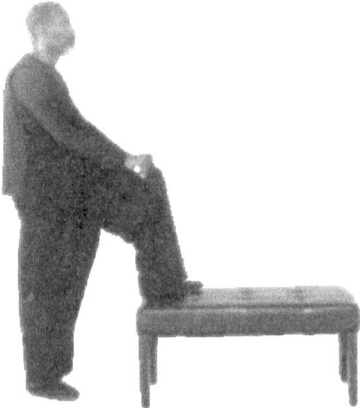

## Left Hamstring & Lower Back One

**1.**

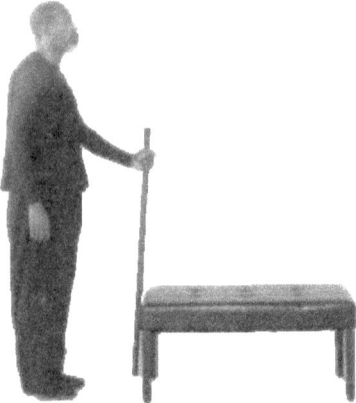

**2.**

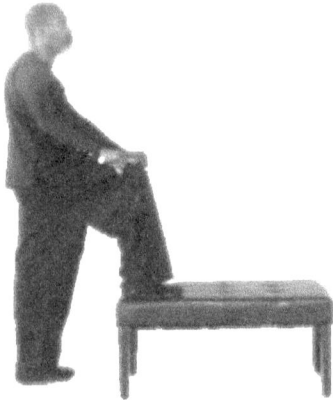

**3.**

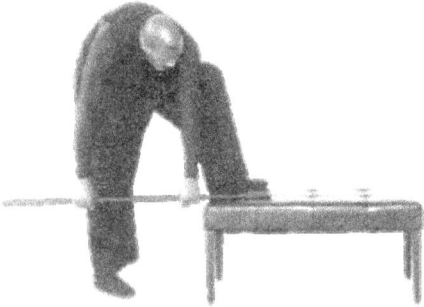

**4.**

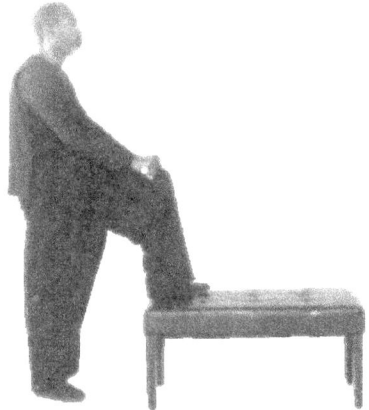

**3.**

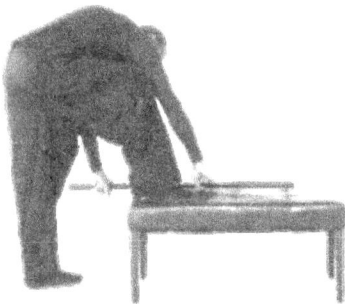

**4.**

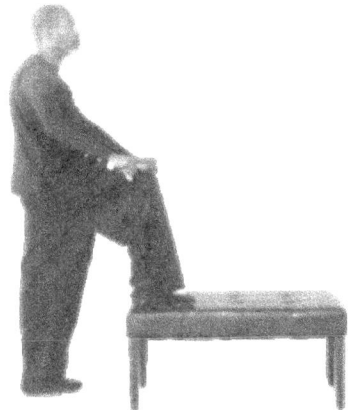

## Right Hamstring & Lower Back Two

1.

2.

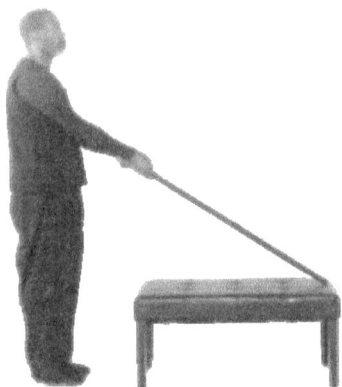
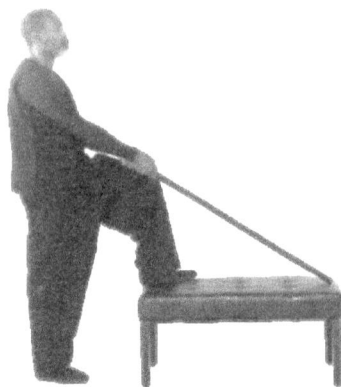

## Left Hamstring & Lower Back Two

1.

2.

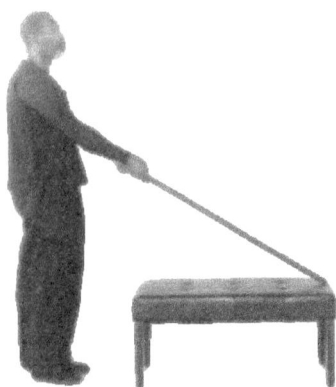
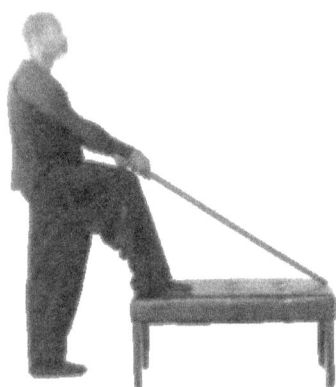

**3.**

**4.**

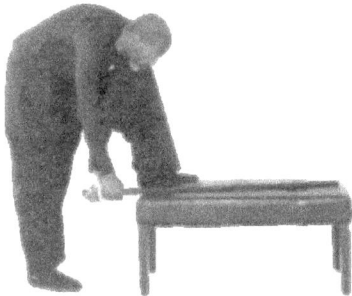
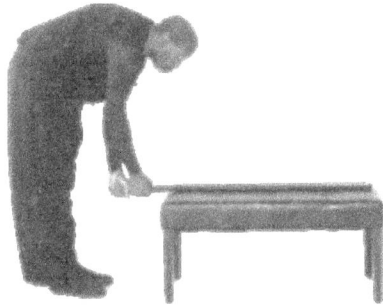

**3.**

**4.**

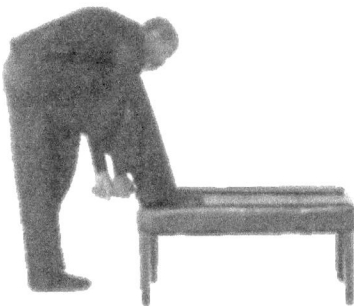
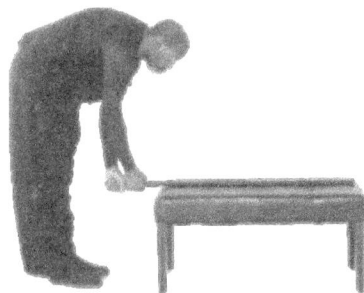

# Left Foot, Instep, & Calf Muscles

## 1.

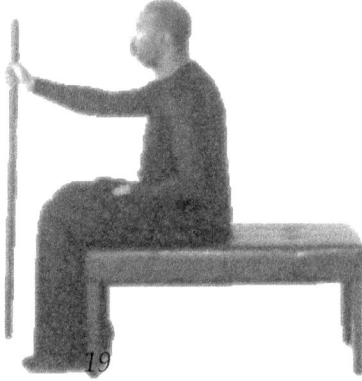

# Right Foot, Instep, & Calf Muscles

## 1.

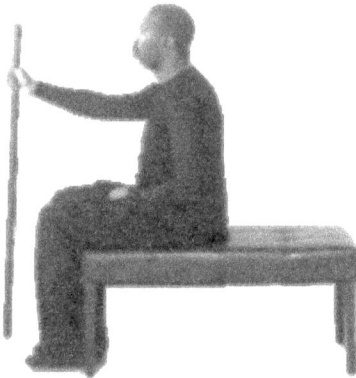

2.

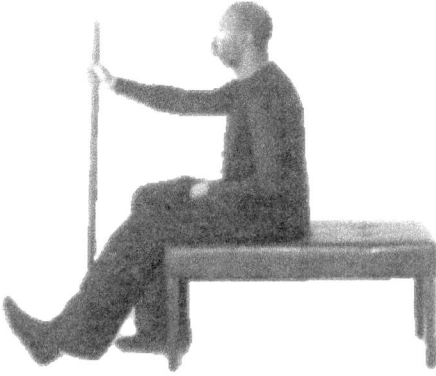

2.

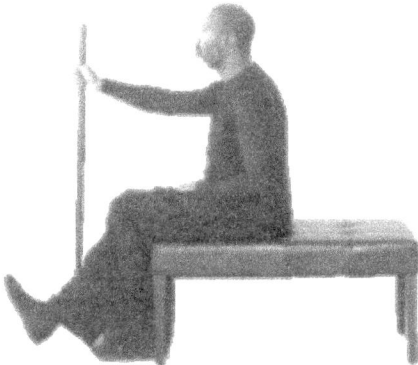

# Inner Thighs

**1.**

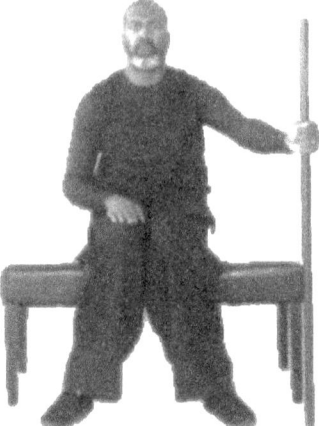

**2.**

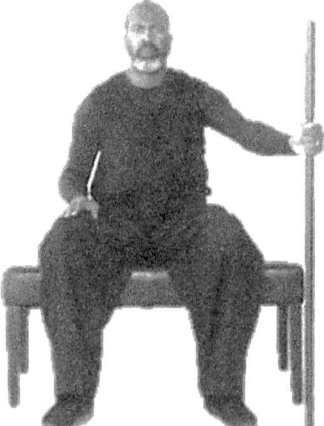

**3.**

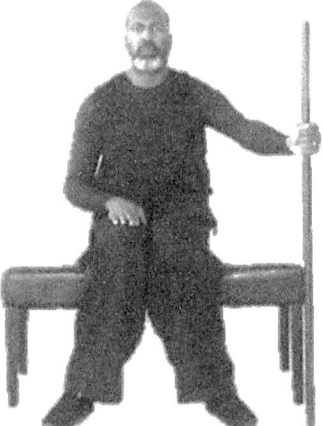

# Mid-Section & Shoulders

1.

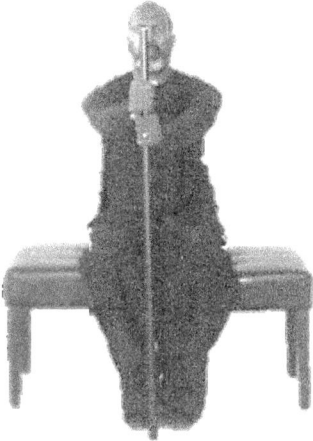

2.

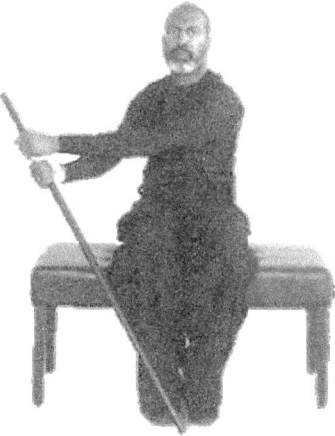

3.

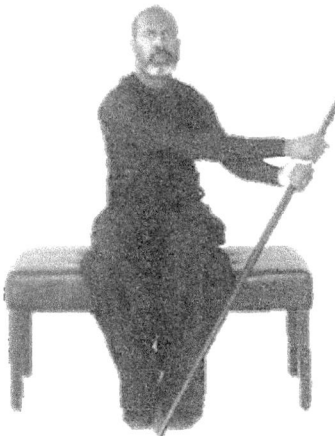

# Mid-Section & Upper Body One

## 1.

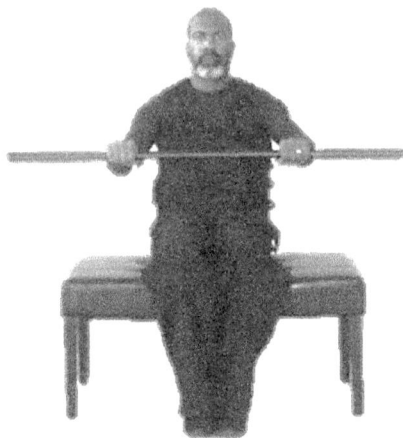

## 2.

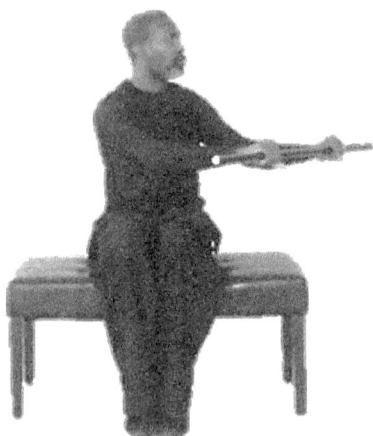

## 3.

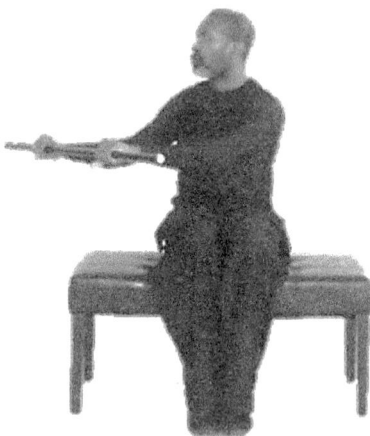

# Mid-Section & Upper Body Two

### 1.

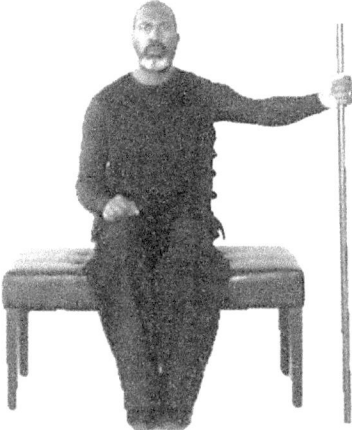

### 2.

### 3.

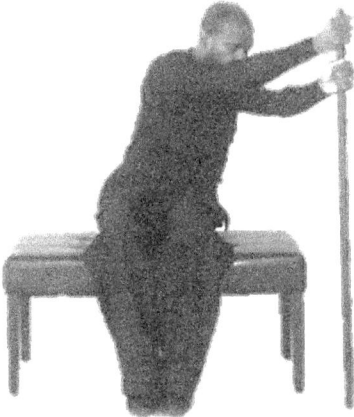
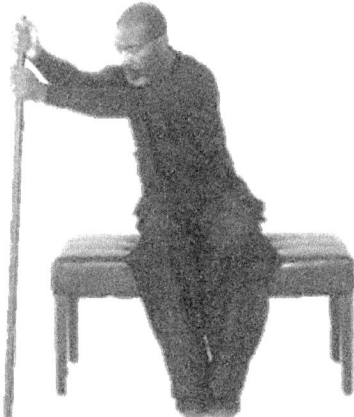

# Mid-Section & Upper Body Three

**1.**

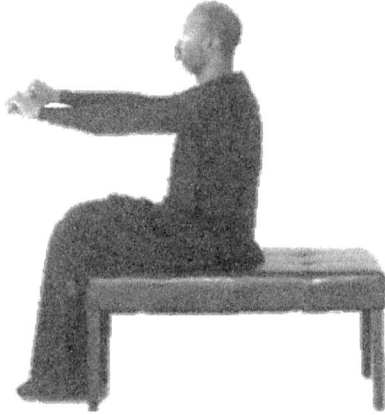

**2.**

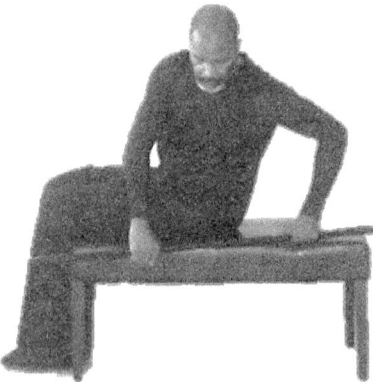

**3.**

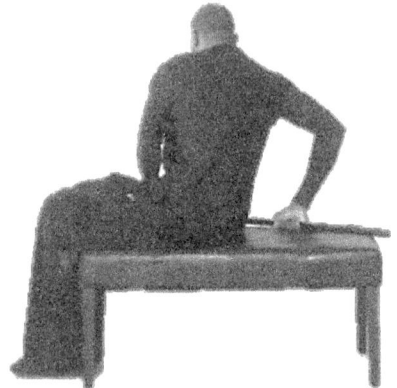

1.

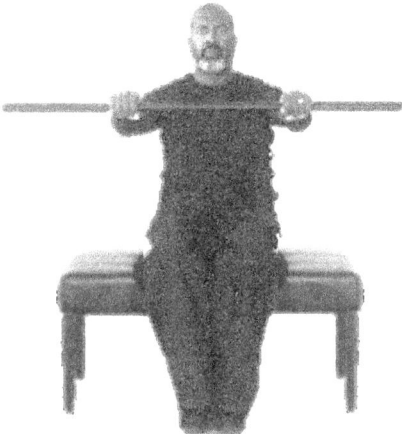

2.

3.

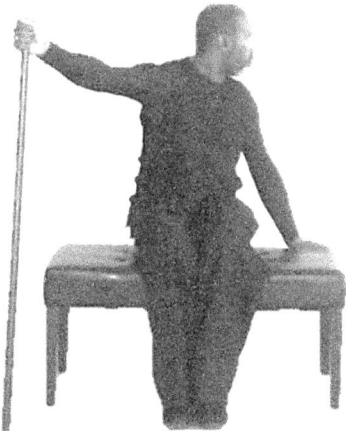
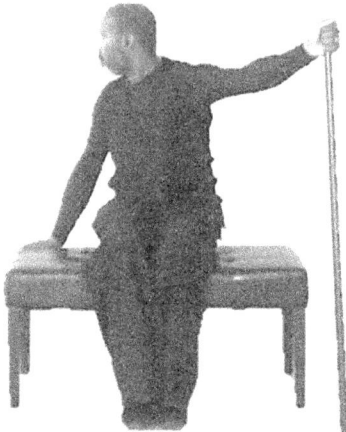

# Left Shoulder, Bicep, & Triceps

**1.**

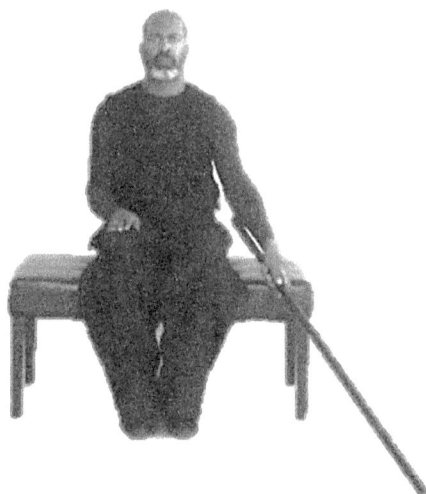

**2.**

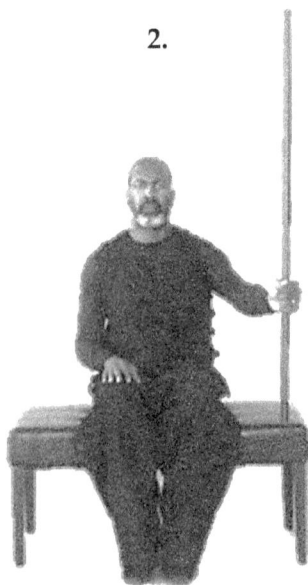

**3.**

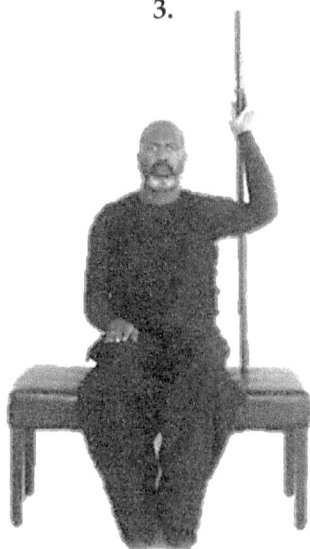

# Right Shoulder, Bicep, & Triceps

**1.**

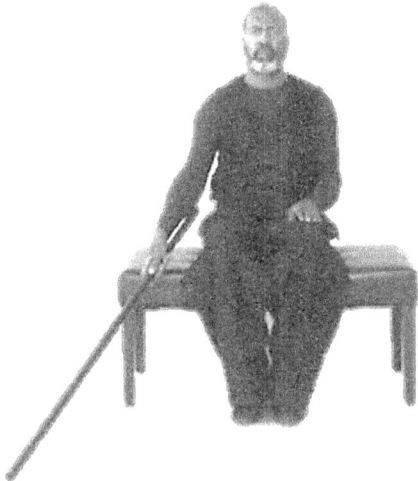

**2.**

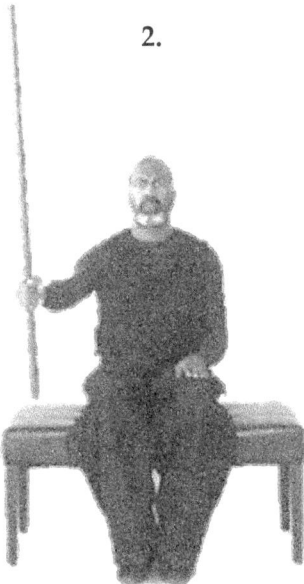

**3.**

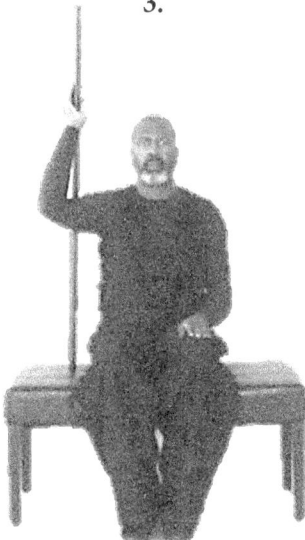

## Lower Back, Ham Strings, & Triceps

**1.**

**2.**

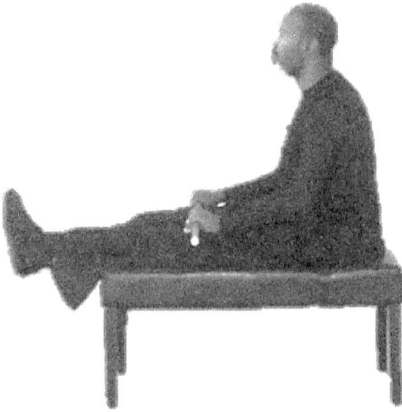
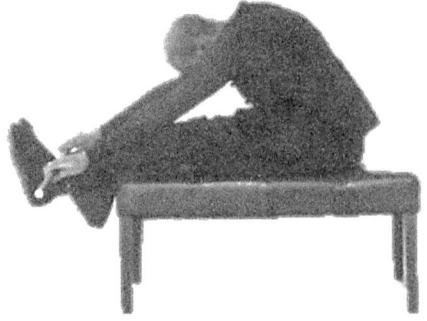

## Lower Back & Left Hamstring / Left Foot

**1.**

**2.**

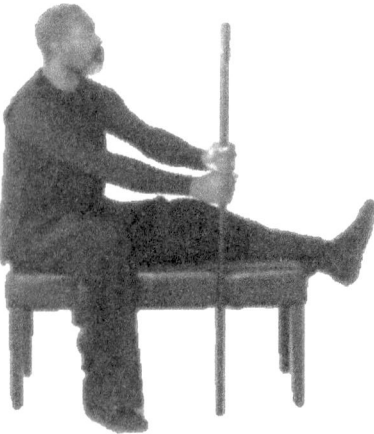
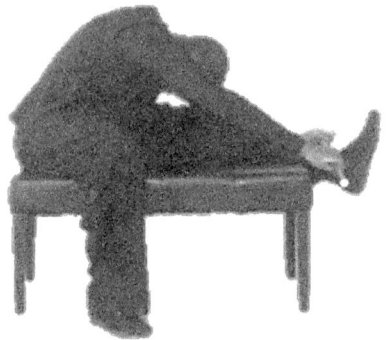

**3.**

**4.**

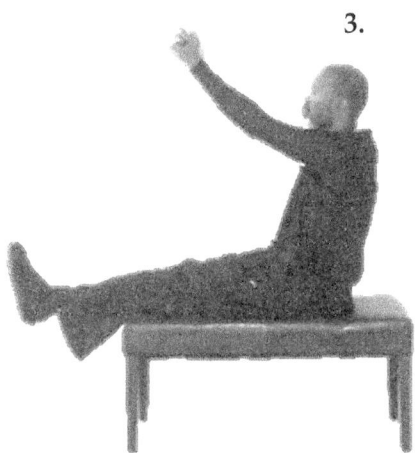

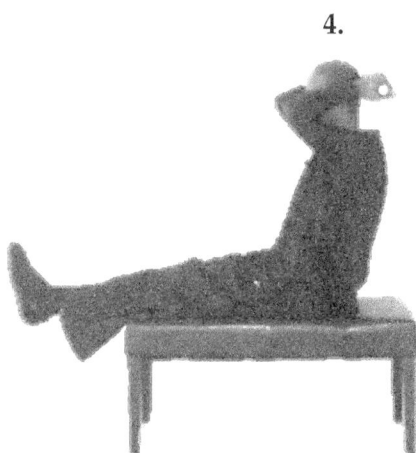

Lower Back & Right Hamstring / Right Foot

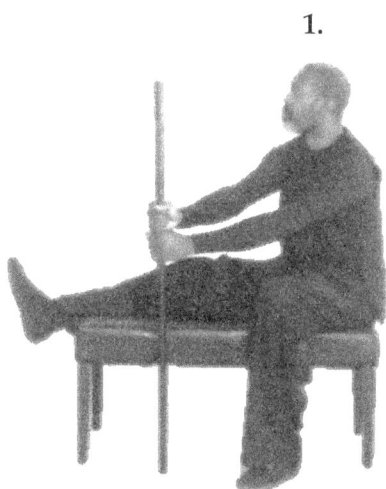

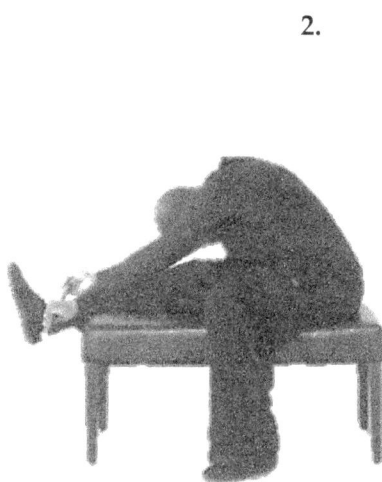

**1.**

**2.**

## Shoulders, Chest & Deltoids

1.

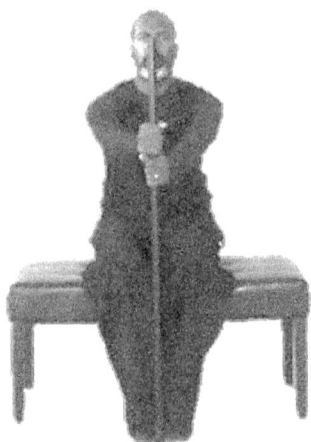

2.

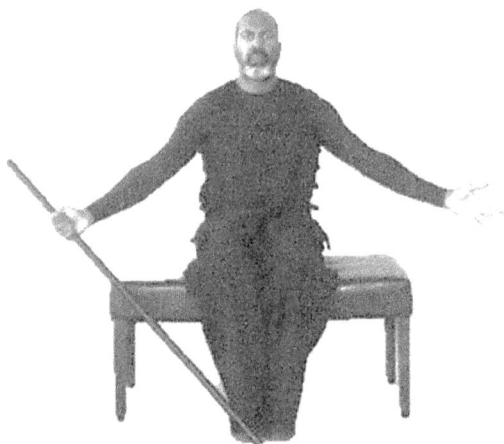

## Right & Left Quadriceps / Shoulders

1.

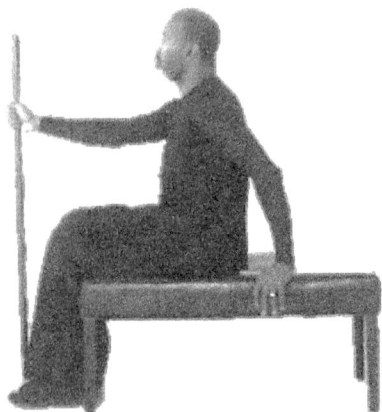

2.

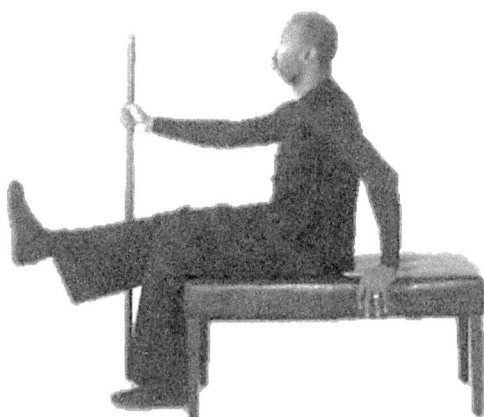

3.

4.

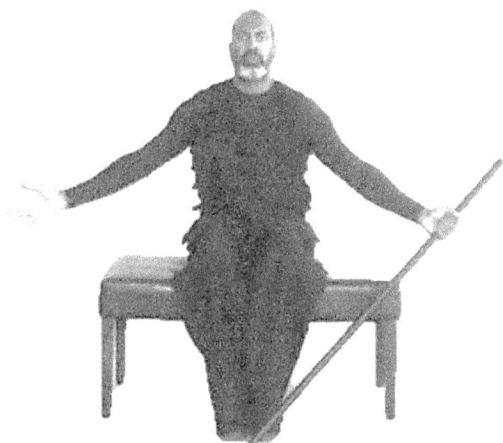

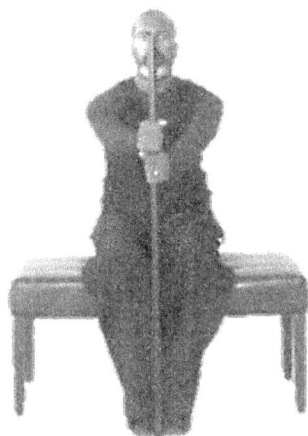

3.

4.

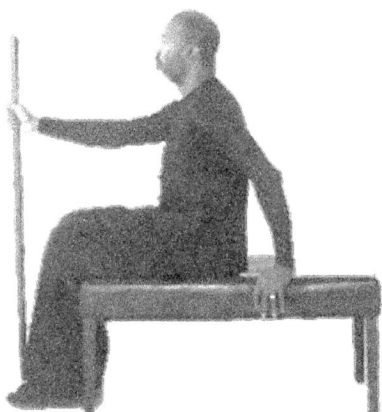

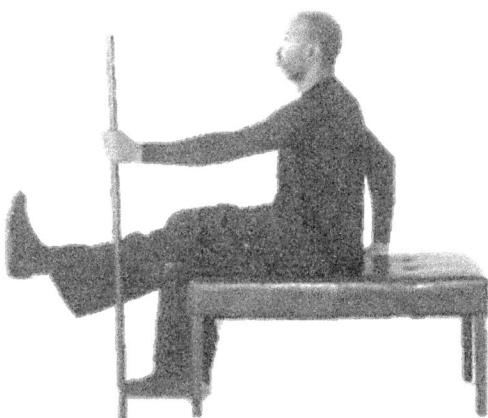

# Shoulders, Chest, & Upper Back

1.

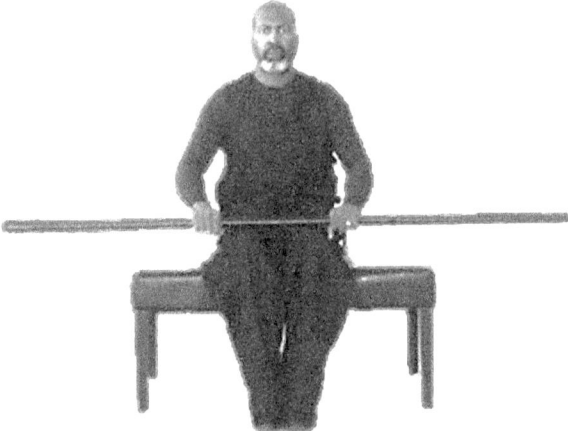

3.

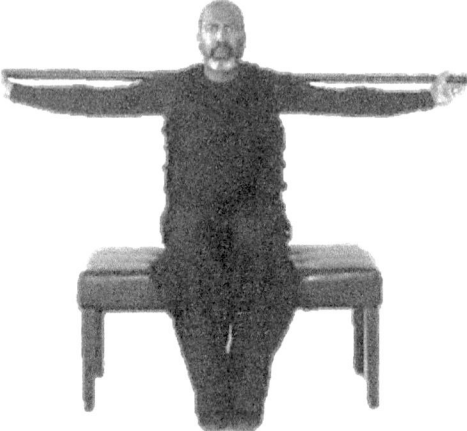

2.

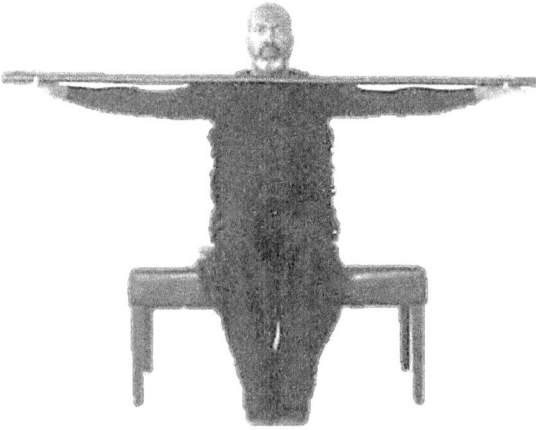

4.

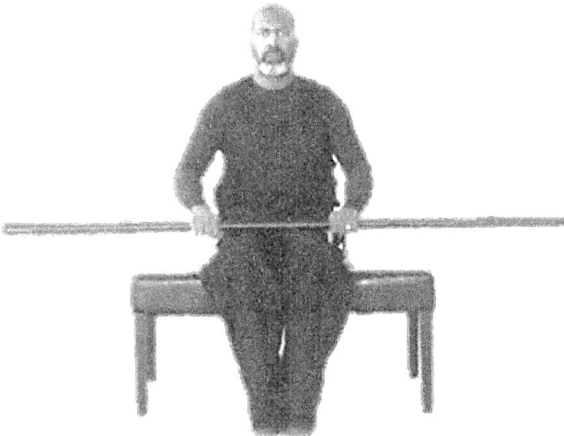

**1.**

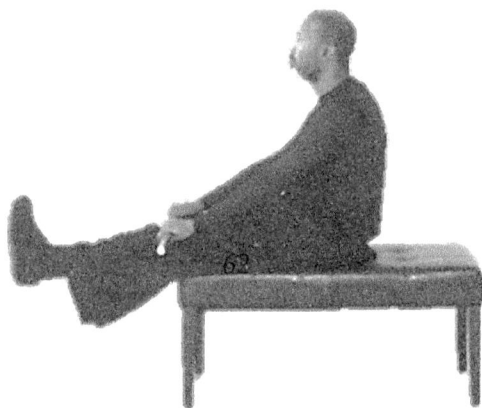

**2.**

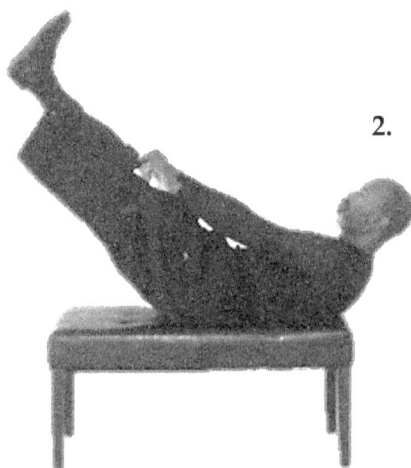

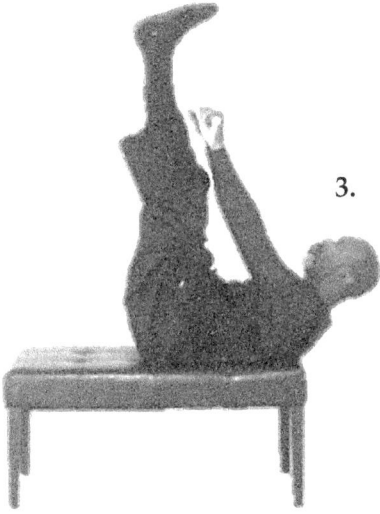

**3.**

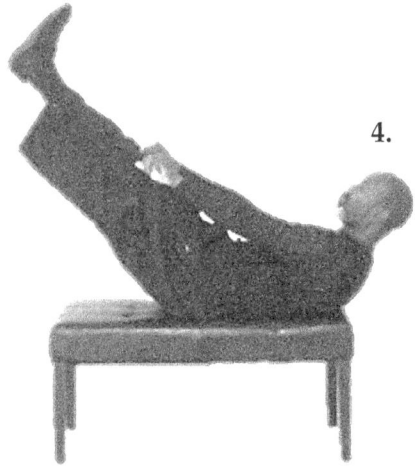

**4.**

**5.**

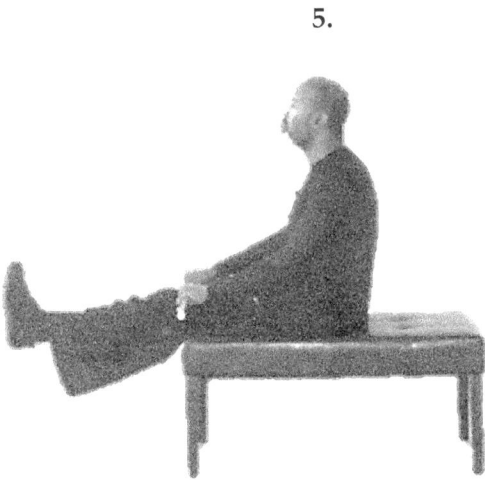

1.

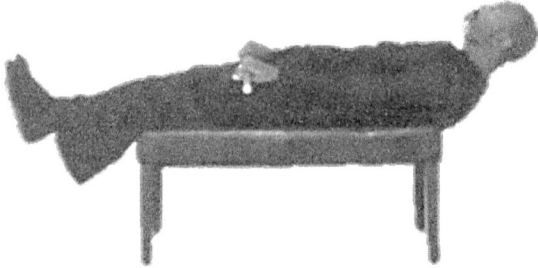

2.

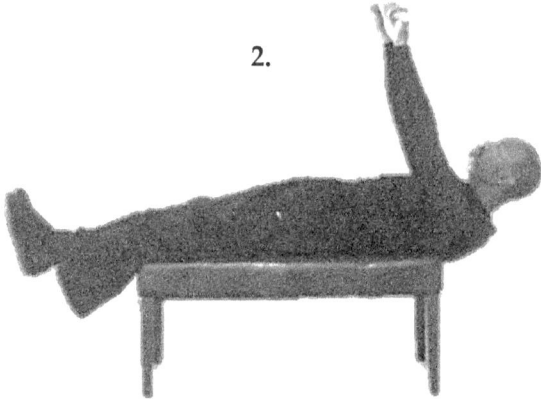

3.

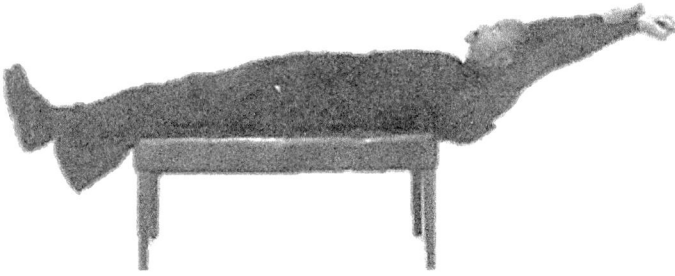

4.

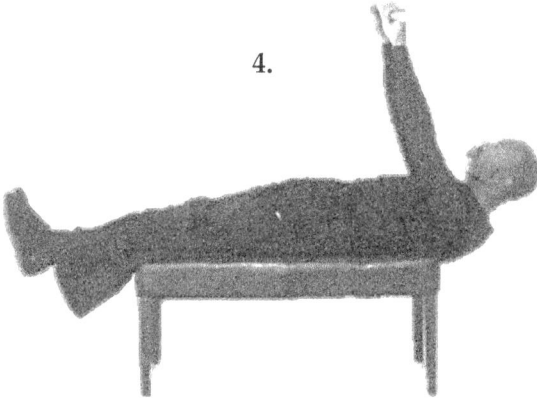

5.

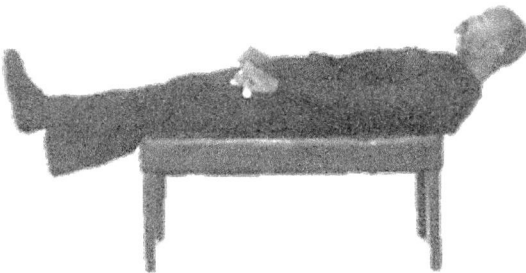

# Midsection & Abdomen

**1.**

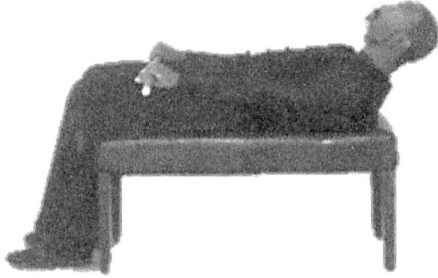

**2.**

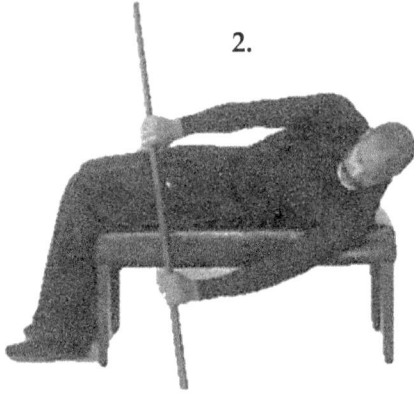

**3.**

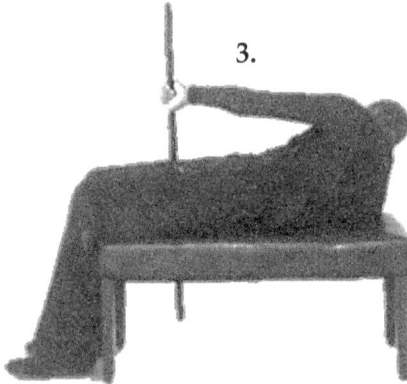

1.

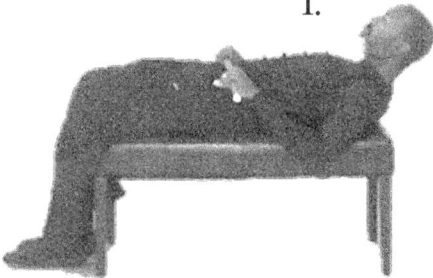

2.

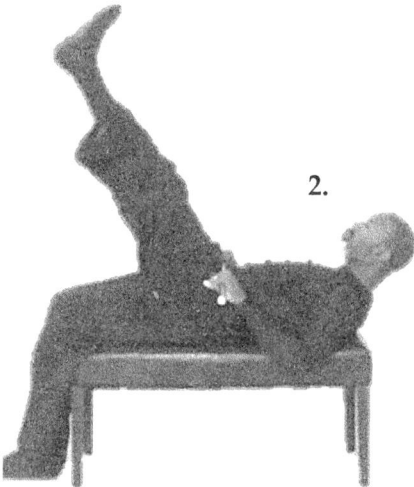

3.

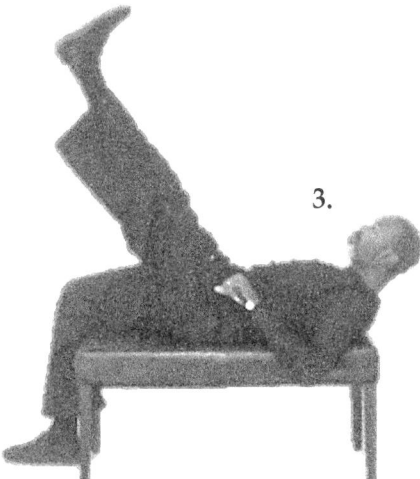

4.

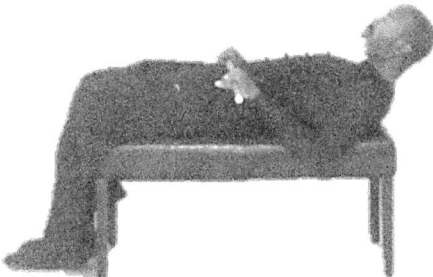

# Bonus Stretching Goal

**1.**

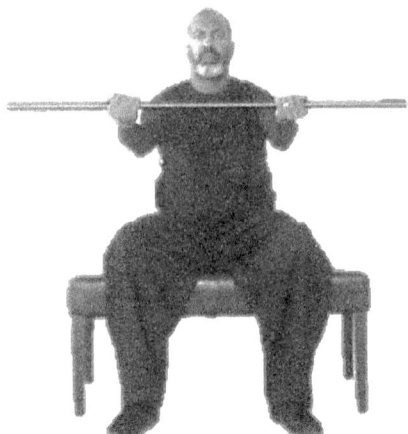

**2.**

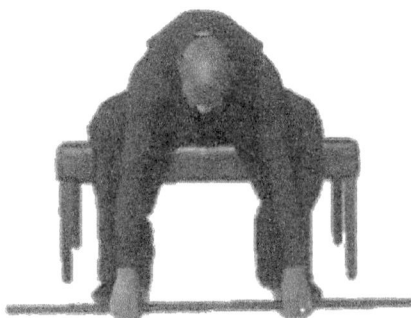

# Lower Back Stretch

**3.**

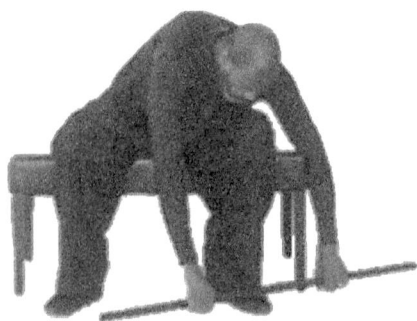

**4.**

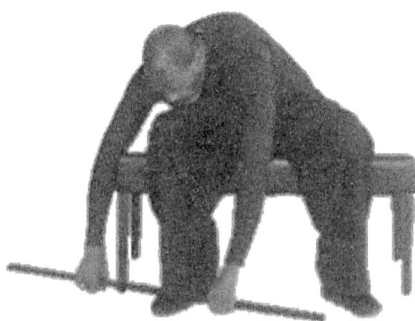

# Authors Note

Doing what is often unnecessary, could very well cause you severe pain, and more frustration. As a rule of thumb, never do more than you can actively handle. The meaning to this, and how it applies is simple. If you feel that you are not ready to advance to the more difficult exercises or segments, then don't.

We are all aware that our muscles have memory. That memory is of what you once did, before you were injured or stricken ill. Knowing this, you are now able to apply the proper form, and function, to the area that has been affected. How many times have you injured yourself, only to reinjure yourself a second time. This is due to poor exercise, and stretching habits. Or, the advice of others who are unaware of your condition, and how to manage it. Thus resulting in a longer waiting period, and recovery time, you are forced to pause your progress.

At the expense of your body, and your future health. Do yourself a favor. Follow the routine your doctors, or physical therapist recommend. Asking yourself what happen, may be too late after it happens.

# Chapter #6 Review

Physical Activity

Muscular Endurance

Flexibility

The Warm - Up

The Cool Down

___

The Twelve Daily Exercises

Stretching

Standing and Sitting Drill

A. Standing (*stretch*)

B. Sitting (*stretch*)

C. Lying Down (*stretch*)

# WU-WEI

## Non - Action

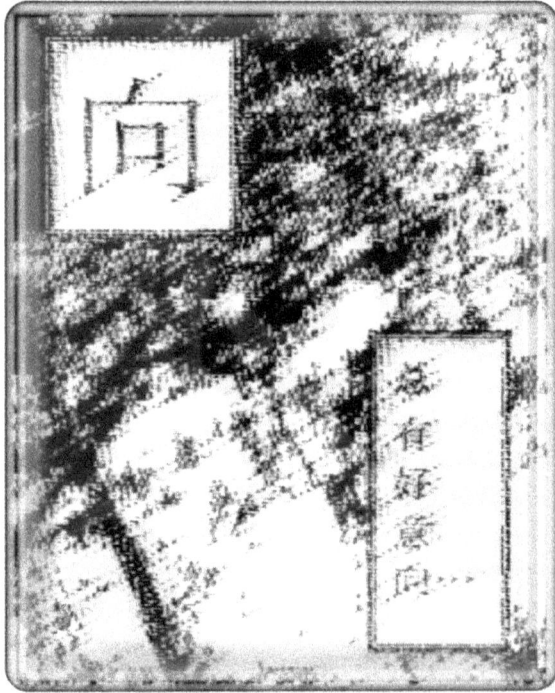

An artist was given a couple of rocks in which to shape.

He was told the form had to be shaped into that of what is.

After a few moments of pondering the shapes and the forms,

the artist decided to leave them as they were naturally formed.

The rocks were already shaped into the form of what is....Wu-Wei

# APPENDIX

---

In the remaining pages you'll find a convenient list of fruits, vegetables, herbs, spices, meats, dairy products etcetera. Each item is broken down into its nutritional value, with a brief explanation of the daily recommended requirements for men and women. Also included is a 30 day exercise chart, and a 12 month weight loss chart to help you keep track of your progress.

# DIET & FITNESS PLAN

*Please consult your doctor, or a qualified nutrition expert, before following this, or any diet, and fitness plan. The Author, nor anyone else involved, will not be held liable for any complications that may occur. The following plan was developed by myself, and approved by my doctors. By following this plan you do so at your own risk, and accept full responsibility of any problems, difficulties, or injuries.*

It doesn't matter how you move in the beginning. What's important is that you are exercising your body to fight against muscular atrophy. You have to be dedicated to this every day. Your joints will lose vital fluid and nutrients within 24 to 48 hours if you are not active every day. By this I mean the ligaments, cartilage, and other soft tissue around your connecting bones. They should be exercised and conditioned daily. This is where water comes into play.

Your muscles, and joints need water to keep them fresh, and replenished daily. You can replenish your minimum requirements of what you need daily with water, and organic fruit juices. If you're like myself and countless others suffering from autoimmune disease, salt can be lethal. Salt will deplete your muscle activity and cause flare ups. I noticed in the beginning of my research that salt would drain, and slow me down physically. We crave salt daily but can learn to avoid consuming excessive amounts. Always watch your salt intake.

**1.** Think positive and find purpose in what you do. Do not feel sorry for yourself anymore. Avoid thinking negatively.

**2.** Exercise every day using slow, and precise movements.

**3.** Try to walk every day. 5 minutes to a max of **30** minutes.

**4.** Your diet must consist of the basic's.

    **a.** No sodas or pops, or whatever you want to call them.

    **b.** No bread of any kind.

    **c.** No red meat, this stuff is poison.

    **d.** No processed foods of any kind.

    **e. NO FAST FOOD EVER**.... Burger King Taco Bell, McDonalds, Pizza Hut, etcetera.

    **f.** No & I mean no sweets . . . . . . .with the exception to dark chocolate.

    **g.** No coffee or artificial stimulates of any kind.

    **h.** No energy drinks.

    **i.** No sugar or sweetener substitutes...

    **j.** No micro wave preheated ready to eat dinners.

**5.** Try to limit the amount of food you eat to 2 or 3 meals a day. When you eat a meal it shouldn't fill you up for the day. Your last meal of the day should be a fruit, or vegetables, not meat.

**6.** Drink at least 1 - 2 liter's a day of water. Start each day by drinking 16 ounces of water to speed up your metabolism, first thing in the morning. **Do not eat, or drink anything after 7:00 p.m....** The only exception to this is to use a **4 - to - 6 oz.** cup of water to take pills in the evening. If your medication requires you to eat before taking it, then do so before **7:00 p.m. in the evening.**

**7.** Eat a high fiber diet. Fruits such as apples, grapes, berry's, and oranges are good sources of fiber.

**8.** Reduce your protein intake of meats to half. This being chicken, turkey, and fish. Poultry should be boneless, no skin. Bake your food to retain vital nutrients, as opposed to boiling. Boiling over a hot oven can inhibit the release of vital vitamins, and minerals. Avoid using grease or cooking oil. Use olive oil, and water. Also use ground lean turkey meat, ground chicken, instead of cow (beef).

**9.** Vegetables should be all natural. Organic if you can find them. None of those store bought meals that are ready to eat.

**10.** Also get plenty of rest, and sleep when you need to. Your body is aware of the change. Your mind has to be aware also.

**11.** Only eat the foods that you cook. This is very hard to do. There are substitutions to this. When eating out only eat at places where you can actually see the menu first. Most importantly look at what's in the food, how it is cooked, and is it in your diet plan of safe foods to eat.

## 12. GET UP, AND MOVE EVERY DAY. NO EXCUSES, NO EXCEPTIONS. KEEP MOVING.

At the start of my diet & fitness plan I weighed,
**256lbs.  6ft. 1in. tall,  48yrs. old.**

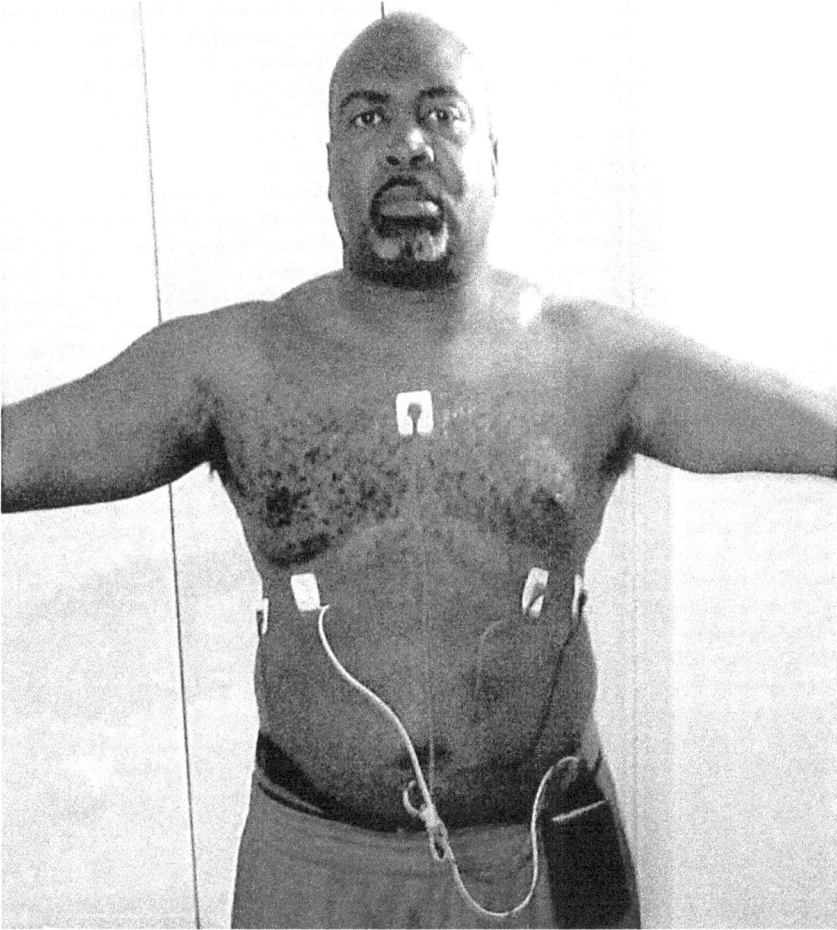

Wearing a Holter Monitor.  Waist 44 inches.

*"The Consummate changes to adapt, and consequently is adaptable to changes unconsciously, that are confirmative, and constructive. Such methods are done at will, and not by the will of force."*

*The Purest* '08

# VITAMINS & MINERALS

Vitamins and minerals are in most of the natural foods we eat. It's better to get them from natural foods.

## Vitamins

**B1 (thiamin)** - spinach, green peas, tomato juice, watermelon, sunflower seeds, lean ham, lean pork chops, and soy milk.

**B2 (riboflavin)** - broccoli, mushrooms, eggs, milk, spinach, liver, oysters, and clams.

**B3 (niacin)** - lean ground beef, chicken breast, tuna spinach, potatoes, tomato juice, liver, and shrimp.

**B6 (pyridoxine)** - bananas, watermelon, tomato juice, broccoli, spinach, acorn squash, potatoes, white rice, and chicken breast.

**B12** - meats, poultry, fish, shellfish, milk, and eggs.

**Biotin** - a common complex vitamin found in egg yolk, and liver.

**Folate** - tomato juice, green beans, broccoli, spinach, asparagus, okra, black-eyed peas, lentils, navy, pinto, and garbanzo beans.

A (retinol) - This can be found in mango, broccoli, butternut squash, carrots, tomato juice, sweet potatoes, pumpkin, and beef liver.

C (ascorbic acid) - spinach, broccoli, red bell peppers, snow peas, tomato juice, kiwi, mango, orange, grapefruit juice, and strawberries.

D - exposure to sunlight, fortified milk, egg yolk, liver, and fatty fish.

E - polyunsaturated plant oils, (soybean, corn, and canola oils), wheat germ, sunflower seeds, tofu, avocado, sweet potatoes, shrimp, and cod.

K - brussels sprouts, leafy green vegetables, spinach, broccoli, cabbage, and liver.

# Minerals

Sodium - salt, soy sauce, bread, milk, and meats.

Chloride - milk, eggs, meat, soy sauce, and salt.

Potassium - potatoes, acorns, squash, artichoke, spinach, broccoli, carrots, green beans, tomato juice, avocado, grapefruit juice, watermelon, banana, strawberries, cod, and milk.

Calcium - milk, yogurt, cheddar cheese, Swiss cheese, tofu, sardines, green beans, spinach, and broccoli.

**Phosphorus** - animal foods, (meats, fish, poultry, eggs, milk).

**Magnesium** - spinach, broccoli, artichokes, green beans, tomato juice, navy beans, pinto beans, black-eyed peas, sunflower seeds, tofu, cashews, and halibut.

**Iron** - artichokes, parsley, spinach, broccoli, green beans, tomato juice, tofu, clams, shrimp, and beef liver.

**Zinc** - spinach, broccoli, green peas, green beans, tomato juice, lentils, oysters, shrimp, crab, turkey (dark meat), lean ham, lean ground beef, lean sirloin steak, plain yogurt, Swiss cheese, tofu, and ricotta cheese.

**Selenium** - seafood, meats, and grain.

**Iodine** - salt, seafood, bread, milk, and cheese.

**Molybdenum** - legumes, and organ meats.

**Copper** - iron, supports formation of hemoglobin, and several enzymes. It's found in various meats and water.

**Manganese** - foods in general.

**Fluoride** - fluorinated drinking water, tea, and seafood.

**Chromium** - vegetable oils, liver, yeast, whole grains, cheese, and nuts.

# Anti-Inflammatory Aids

**Turmeric** - anti-inflammatory compound also known as, curcuma longa. Also to include garlic, cinnamon, and ginger for anti-inflammatory value.

**Salmon** - one of the highest as an anti-inflammatory aid, with omega-3 fatty acids, sardines, halibut, mackerel, black cod, tuna, herring, and anchovies.

**Olive Oil** - jam-packed with powerful antioxidants. Also good for cooking and baking.

**Water** - has a minimum amount of anti-inflammatory power, along with green tea, and black tea. Best source to use when replenishing sore aching muscles...

Nature has given us some incredible foods that can be used to help fight against autoimmune disease, or chronic inflammatory disorders. One of the major causes of inflammation in our bodies other than disease is the food we eat. The right foods can help solve some of the problems of inflammation. By eating such foods as those mentioned you can fight back against inflammation. Other foods that help fight inflammation are, oranges, walnuts, tuna, ginger, garlic, and strawberries.

# Recommended Daily Amount
## Vitamin & Mineral Charts

**milligrams** (*mg*), **micrograms** (*mcg*)
*1,000 mcg = 1 mg, & International Units (IU)*

| VITAMINS | Women 18 & Older | Men 18 & Older |
|---|---|---|
| A | 700 mcg | 900 mcg |
| B1 | 1.1 mg | 1.2 mg |
| B2 | 1.1 mg | 1.3 mg |
| B3 | 14 mg | 16 mg |
| B6 | 1.3 mg | 1.3 mg |
| B12 | 2.4 mcg | 2.4 mcg |
| C | 75 mg | 90 mg |
| D | 5 mcg | 5 mcg |
| E | 15 mcg | 15 mcg |
| K | 90 mcg | 120 mcg |
| Folate | 400 mcg | 400 mcg |
| Biotin | 30 mcg | 30 mcg |

1 *mg* = **1 milligram** = 1/1,000 of a **gram**

1 *μg* = 1 *mcg* = **1 microgram** = 1/1,000,000 of a **gram**

| MINERALS | Women 18 & Older | Men 18 & Older |
|---|---|---|
| Sodium | 500 mg | 500 mg |
| Potassium | 2000 mg | 2000 mg |
| Calcium | 800 mg | 800 mg |
| Phosphorus | 700 mg | 700 mg |
| Magnesium | 320 mg | 420 mg |
| Iron | 15mg | 10mg |
| Zinc | 12mg | 15mg |
| Selenium | 55mcg | 70mcg |
| Iodine | 150 mcg | 150 mcg |
| Molybdenum | 45mcg | 45mcg |
| Copper | 1.5-3.0 mg | 1.5-3.0 mg |
| Manganese | 2.5 mg | 2.5 mg |
| Chromium | 50-200 mcg | 50-200 mcg |

# Herbs & Spices

**Fennel** – fennel bulb leaves can be used as an herb. Raw fennel is a good source of vitamin C, folate, phosphorus, calcium, magnesium, potassium, manganese iron, copper, and vitamin B3 (niacin). It is also an antioxidant with anti-inflammatory properties.

**Basil** – vitamin A, magnesium, iron, potassium, calcium, vitamin C. It also has anti-inflammatory properties, and stimulates cardiovascular health.

**Ginger** – magnesium, copper, potassium, manganese, and vitamin B6 (pyridoxine).

**Coriander** - known to be anti-inflammatory, and cholesterol lowering. Increases HDL (the "good" cholesterol). Coriander is a good source of dietary fiber, manganese, iron, and magnesium.

**Sage** – antioxidant and anti-inflammatory properties. Sage has dietary fiber, vitamin A (carotenoid), calcium, and iron.

**Thyme** – vitamin K, iron, manganese, calcium, and dietary fiber.

**Cloves** – vitamin K, dietary fiber, vitamin C, manganese, and a good source of omega-3 fatty acids. Anti-inflammatory properties as well.

**Garlic** – manganese, vitamin B6 (pyridoxine), vitamin C, selenium, calcium, phosphorus, vitamin B1 (thiamin), copper, and protein.

**Mustard Seeds** – selenium, omega-3 fatty acids, phosphorus, manganese, magnesium, dietary fiber, iron, calcium, protein, vitamin B3 (niacin), and zinc. Known to have anti-inflammatory properties.

**Oregano** – vitamin K, manganese, iron, dietary fiber, omega-3 fatty acids, calcium, vitamin A, and vitamin C. The highest amount of antioxidant activity.

**Cumin** – iron, manganese. Also can promote healthy immune functions, good digestion. Good as a anti - inflammatory aide .

**Dill** - iron, manganese, and calcium. Could possibly help guard against free-radical damage, and has anti-bacterial properties.

# Nuts & Seeds

**Almonds** – vitamin E, manganese, magnesium, copper, vitamin B2 (riboflavin), and phosphorus. Almonds have concentrated amounts of protein.

**Sunflower Seeds** – anti-inflammatory, and cardiovascular benefits, lower cholesterol. Excellent source of vitamin E, linoleic acid (an essential fatty acid), dietary fiber, protein, and minerals such as magnesium, and selenium.

**Pumpkin Seeds** - good source of the essential fatty acids, potassium, phosphorous, magnesium, manganese, zinc, iron, and copper, protein, and vitamin K.

**Flaxseeds** – folate, vitamin B6 (pyridoxine), magnesium, phosphorous, and copper, and lignan phytonutrients. Excellent source of omega-3 fatty acids. Has anti-inflammatory properties, as well as bone protection.

**Peanuts** – folic acid, vitamin B3 (niacin), folate, copper, manganese, and protein.

**Cashews** – high in antioxidants, and a very low fat content compared to other nuts; 75 percent of its fat is unsaturated fatty acids. Also have monounsaturated fats, copper, and a good source of magnesium and phosphorous.

**Sesame Seeds** – manganese, and copper, calcium, magnesium, iron, phosphorous, vitamin B1 (thiamin), zinc, dietary fiber, and powerful antioxidants called lignan, and help provide relief for rheumatoid arthritis, and support vascular respiratory health.

**Walnuts** – omega-3 essential fatty acids, manganese, and copper. Good source of healthy monounsaturated fats. Benefit your cardiovascular system. Aid in protecting bone health, and help prevent gallstones. Melatonin, which helps regulate sleep.

# HEALTHY FOODS

## Eggs & Dairy

| | |
|---|---|
| Goats Milk | Milk 2% |
| Eggs<br>Organically fed chickens | Cheese<br>low-fat |
| Greek Yogurt<br>plain no sugar | |

## Grains

| | |
|---|---|
| Barley | Millet |
| Buckwheat | Brown Rice |
| Oats | Corn |
| Quinoa | Rye |
| Whole Wheat | Spelt |

# Meats

| | |
|---|---|
| **Chicken** / free roaming | **Turkey** / free roaming |
| Lamb | **Beef** Organically fed |
| Venison | |

# Beans & Legumes

| | |
|---|---|
| Black Beans | Dried Peas |
| Garbanzo Beans (chickpeas) | Kidney Beans |
| Lentils | Lima Beans |
| Miso | Navy Beans |
| Pinto Beans | Soybeans |
| Black Eyed Peas | Green Beans |
| NA | NA |

# Vegetables

| | | | |
|---|---|---|---|
| Asparagus | Avocados | Beets | Bell Peppers |
| Broccoli | Brussels Sprouts | Cabbage | Carrots |
| Cauliflower | Celery | Collard Greens | Cucumbers |
| Eggplant | Fennel | Garlic | Green Beans |
| Green Peas | Kale | Leeks | Mushrooms |
| Mustard Greens | Olives | Onions | Potatoes |
| Romaine Lettuce | Sea Vegetables | Spinach | Squash, Summer |
| Sweet Potatoes | Swiss Chard | Tomatoes | Turnip Greens |

# Sea Foods

| | | |
|---|---|---|
| Cod & Tuna | Salmon | Sardines |
| Halibut | Shrimp | Scallops |

# Fruits

| Apples | Apricots | Bananas | Cranberries |
|--------|----------|---------|-------------|
| Blueberries | Cantaloupe | Figs | Grapefruit |
| Grapes | Kiwifruit | Lemon | Limes |
| Oranges | Papaya | Pears | Raisins |
| Pineapple | Prunes | Plums | Raspberries |
| Strawberries | | Watermelon | |

# Calorie Consumption

**1.** Adults average between **2,000** and **3,000** calories a day.

**2.** Women need fewer calories. This includes less active people.

**3.** Men need more calories. This includes more active people.

If you are eating the recommended daily amount of calories per day, and following your daily plan or fitness régime, your weight should vary between two to five pounds a day. You should also add in the amount of water you drink as well. Your calorie consumption should be between, **40** to **50** percent from carbohydrates, **30** percent from fat, and **20** to **30** percent from protein. Make it a daily practice to include carbohydrates, fat, protein, and fiber in each meal.

# Carbohydrates

**1.** Based on the recommended daily amount for calorie consumption, an adult women should consume between 160 to 200 grams of carbohydrates a day.

**2.** Based on the recommended daily amount for calorie consumption, an adult man should consume between 240 to 300 grams of carbohydrates a day.

**3.** Reduce or cut out the amount of processed foods you eat.

**4.** Reduce or cut out the amount of wheat flour and sugar. This also includes bread. Avoid packaged snack foods.

**5.** Eat more whole grains like brown rice.

# Fat

**1.** Based on the recommended daily amount for calorie consumption, 600 calories a day should come from fat. Or about 67 grams.

**2.** Use extra-virgin olive oil to cook your foods. Make it a habit to avoid using, sunflower oils, corn oil, cottonseed oil, and mixed vegetable oils.

**3.** Last but not least, avoid margarine, and vegetable shortening, as a substitute for cooking ingredients.

# Protein

**1.** Based on the recommended daily amount for calorie consumption , your daily intake of protein should be between **80** and **120** grams. You should be eating small amounts of protein if you have a liver or kidney problem. Especially if you have trouble with autoimmune diseases, or an allergy problem.

**2.** Cut or reduce the amount of animal protein. With the exceptions of fish and high quality natural cheese. You can still enjoy yogurt daily. Greek Yogurt is the best choice.

**3.** The more vegetable protein the better, especially from beans, and soybeans as these are a reasonable addition.

# Fiber

Based on the recommended daily amount for calorie consumption, you should eat **40** grams of fiber a day. Fruits, berries, vegetables, and whole grains.

| Carbohydrates | 240 - 300 Grams = to **Men** |
| Carbohydrates | 160 - 200 Grams = to **Women** |
| Proteins | 80 - 120 Grams |
| Fats | 67 Grams |

# Metabolism Types

| Type A - *(Protein)* | |
|---|---|
| 50% | Protein |
| 30% | Fats |
| 20% | Carbs |

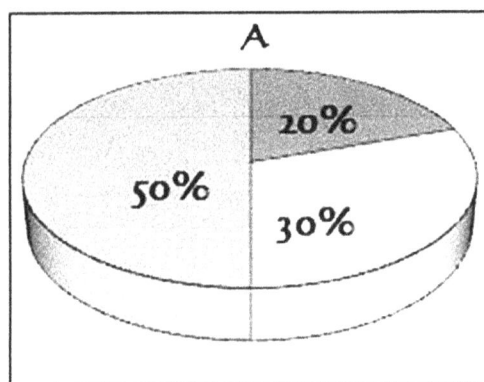

A

20%
50%
30%

| Type B - *(Carbs)* | |
|---|---|
| 20% | Protein |
| 10% | Fats |
| 70% | Carbs |

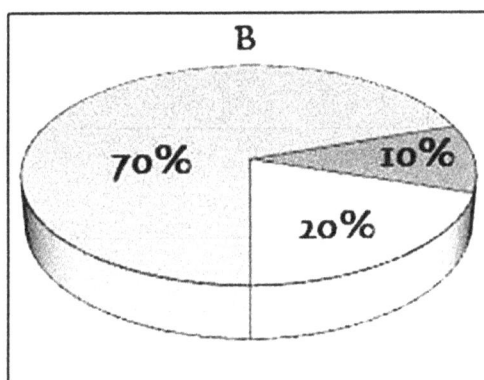

B

70%
10%
20%

| Type C - *(Mixed)* | |
|---|---|
| 33% | Protein |
| 33% | Fats |
| 33% | Carbs |

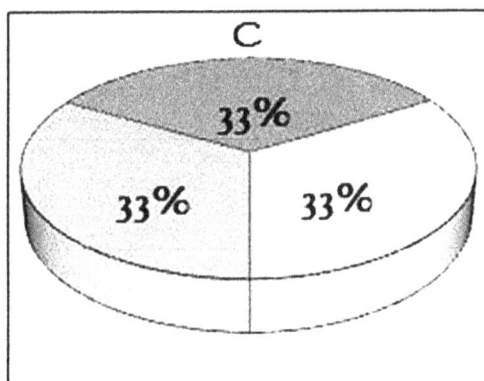

C

33%
33%
33%

# Protein Types

A person with a protein dominant system craves salty, or fatty foods. This individual thrives on a high-protein diet, and doesn't do well on vegetarian or low-fat diets.

1. Have energy extremes.
2. Can be very wired or lethargic.
3. Are anxious and edgy at times.

# Carb Types

A person with a carb dominant system is the exact opposite of the protein dominant type. Carb types function better on whole grains, fruits, and vegetables.

1. Requires less protein.
2. Favors a vegetarian diet.
3. Tends to have a weaker appetite.
4. Has a craving for sweets.

# Mixed Types

A person with a mixed-type system craves sweet foods, carbs, and fatty salty foods. The mixed type has no major energy extremes, but their metabolism is balanced with, carbohydrates, proteins, and fats. They tolerate low-fat, and high-fat proteins. Mixed types require equal portions of meats, dairy, fish, whole grains, legumes or other starches. Mixed types also need fruits, and vegetables each day.

# Metabolic Body Types

Knowing your Metabolic type can help you lose weight.

| | |
|---|---|
| Android | 1. Broad shoulders.<br><br>2. Large rib cage.<br><br>3. Narrow pelvis and hips. |
| Gynaeoid | 1. Curvaceous body.<br><br>2. Small waist & wide hips.<br><br>3. Small to medium shoulders. |
| Thyroid | 1. Slender face.<br><br>2. Long limbs, hands, fingers.<br><br>3. Narrow bones. |
| Lymphatic | 1. Slow metabolism.<br><br>2. Gain weight easy.<br><br>3. Baby-doll body. |

# Anti - Inflammatory Foods

Aids the body in fighting off inflammation.

| | | |
|---|---|---|
| Blue Berries | Almonds | Artichokes |
| Avocado | Basil | Raspberries |
| Buck Wheat | Cabbage | Carrots |
| Cauliflower | Celery | Chives |
| Coconut Oil | Cumin Seeds | Oranges |
| Garlic | Cherries | Apples |
| Lemon | Lettuce | Sweet Potato |
| Onion | Black Berries | Green Beans |
| Rutabaga | Straw Berries | Broccoli |
| Spinach | Olives | Cherries |
| Ginger | Turnips | Papaya |
| White Radish | Oregano | Parsley |

# Water Rich Foods
Contains a high amount of water.

| | |
|---|---|
| Cucumber 96% | Water Melon 96% |
| Pineapple 95% | Broccoli 95% |
| Tomato 94% | Blue Berries 95% |
| Celery 94% | Cantaloupe 93% |
| Grape Fruit 92% | Pears 90% |

# Alkaline Rich Foods
Helps prevent the build-up of lactic acid.

| | |
|---|---|
| Lemons pH 9.0 | Watermelon pH 9.0 |
| Grapes pH 8.0 | Cayenne pH 8.5 |
| Banana pH 8.0 | Fruit Juices pH 8.5 |
| Apples pH 8.0 | N/A |

# Protein Rich Foods

Protein can be found in foods other than meat.

| Split Peas | Baked Potato | Green Peas |
|---|---|---|
| Spinach | Artichokes | Beets |
| Anchovies | Peppers | Broccoli |
| Papaya | Almond Nuts | Banana |
| Peanut Butter | Soy Beans | Pumpkin Seeds |
| Sunflower Seeds | Cheese | N/A |

# Serotonin Rich Foods

A healthy diet lifts your mood, and raises energy levels.

| Cayenne Peppers | Water |
|---|---|
| Almonds | Oats |
| Walnuts | Greens |
| Bananas | Vegetable Smoothies |

# Fiber Rich Foods

Fiber cleans the body, and stimulates digestion.

| | | |
|---|---|---|
| Lima Beans | Adzuki Beans | Black Beans |
| Lentils | Kidney Beans | Navy Beans |
| Pinto Beans | Raspberries | Blue Berries |
| Straw Berries | Boysenberries | Blackberries |
| Popcorn | Oats | Wild Rice |
| Brown Rice | Black Eye Peas | Split Peas |
| Green Peas | Turnip Greens | Mustard Greens |
| Collard Greens | Spinach | Almonds |
| Pistachios | Cashews | Peanuts |
| Walnuts | Flaxseed | Squash |
| Kale | Cauliflower | Banana |
| Pear | Orange | Apple |

# Carbohydrate Rich Foods

Eat more whole grains like brown rice.

| | | |
|---|---|---|
| Bagel | Oatmeal | Apples |
| Yogurt | Artichoke | Corn |
| Carrots | Beans | Muffins |
| Pomegranate | Cantaloupe | Broccoli |
| Peaches | Apricot | Brown Rice |

# Fatty Rich Foods

Eat more omega 3 foods.

| | | |
|---|---|---|
| Tofu | Scallops | Halibut |
| Shrimp | Soybeans | Flax Seed |
| Cloves | Walnuts | Salmon |
| Tuna | Collard Greens | Sardines |
| Winter Squash | Spinach | Turnip Greens |

# CONVERSION CHARTS

## Metric Capacity

| | |
|---|---|
| 1 ml | = less than, 1/4 teaspoon |
| 2 ml | = less than, 1/2 teaspoon |
| 5 ml | = 1 teaspoon |
| 15 ml | = 1 tablespoon |
| 25 ml | = 1 T. plus 2 tsp. |
| 50 ml | = 1/4 c. minus 2 tsp. |
| 125 ml | = 1/2 c. plus 1 1/2 tsp. |
| 250 ml | = 1 c. plus 1 T. |
| 500 ml | = 1 pt. plus 2 T. |
| 1 L | = 1 qt. plus 1/4 c. |

## Metric Weight

| | |
|---|---|
| 30 g | = 1 oz. plus a lg. pinch |
| 125 g | = 1/4 lb. plus 1/4 oz. |
| 250 g | = 1/2 lb. plus less than 1 oz. |
| 500 g | = 1 lb. plus 1 2/3 oz. |
| 0.750 kg | = 1 1/2 lbs. plus 2 1/2 oz. |
| 1 kg | = 2 lbs. plus 3 1/2 oz. |

# Metric Tables

| Measure | Equivalent | Metric (ML) |
|---|---|---|
| 1 tablespoon | 3 teaspoons | 14.8 milliliters |
| 2 tablespoons | 1 ounce | 29.6 milliliters |
| 1 jigger | 1 ½ ounces | 44.4 milliliters |
| ¼ cup | 4 tablespoons | 59.2 milliliters |
| 1/3 cup | 5 tablespoons plus 1 teaspoon | 78.9 milliliters |
| ½ cup | 8 tablespoons | 118.4 milliliters |
| 1 cup | 16 tablespoons | 236.8 milliliters |
| 1 pint | 2 cups | 473.6 milliliters |
| 1 quart | 4 cups | 947.2 milliliters |
| 1 liter | 4 cups plus 3 tablespoons | 1000.0 milliliters |
| 1 ounce (dry) | 2 tablespoons | 28.35 grams |
| 1 pound | 16 ounces | 453.59 grams |
| 2.21 pounds | 35.3 ounces | 1.00 kilogram |

# Liquid Measures

| Imperial | Metric |
|---|---|
| 1 teaspoon | 5 ml |
| 1 tablespoon | 15 ml |
| 2 fluid ounces (1/4 cup) | 62.5 ml |
| 4 fluid ounces (1/2 cup) | 125 ml |
| 8 fluid ounces (1 cup) | 250 ml |
| 1 pint (16 oz.) | 500 ml |

# Equivalent Estimates I

| | |
|---|---|
| Vitamin A - 1 micro gram | 3.33 IU |
| Vitamin D - 1 microgram | 40 IU |
| 28 grams | 1 ounces |
| 100 grams | 3.5 ounces |
| 454 grams | 1 pound |
| 1 tsp. | 5 milliliters |
| 1 quart | 1 liter |

# Equivalent Estimates II

| Spoons & Cups | Ounces | Grams |
|---|---|---|
| 1 tablespoon | ¼ ounce | 8.75 grams |
| ¼ cup (4 Tbsp.) | 1 ¼ ounces | 35 grams |
| ⅓ cup (5 Tbsp.) | 1 ½ ounces | 45 grams |
| ½ cup | 2 ½ ounces | 70 grams |
| 2/3 cup | 3 ¼ ounces | 90 grams |
| ¾ cup | 3 ½ ounces | 105 grams |
| 1 cup | 5 ounces | 140 grams |
| 1 ½ cups | 7 ½ ounces | 210 grams |
| 2 cups | 10 ounces | 280 grams |
| 2 ½ cups | 16 ounces (1 pound) | 490 grams |
| 1 cubic centimeter | = 0.27 fluid dram | N/A |
| 1 liter | = 1.06 liquid quarts | |

At the end of my diet & fitness plan I weighed,
**186 lbs. 6ft. 1in. tall, 49yrs. old.**

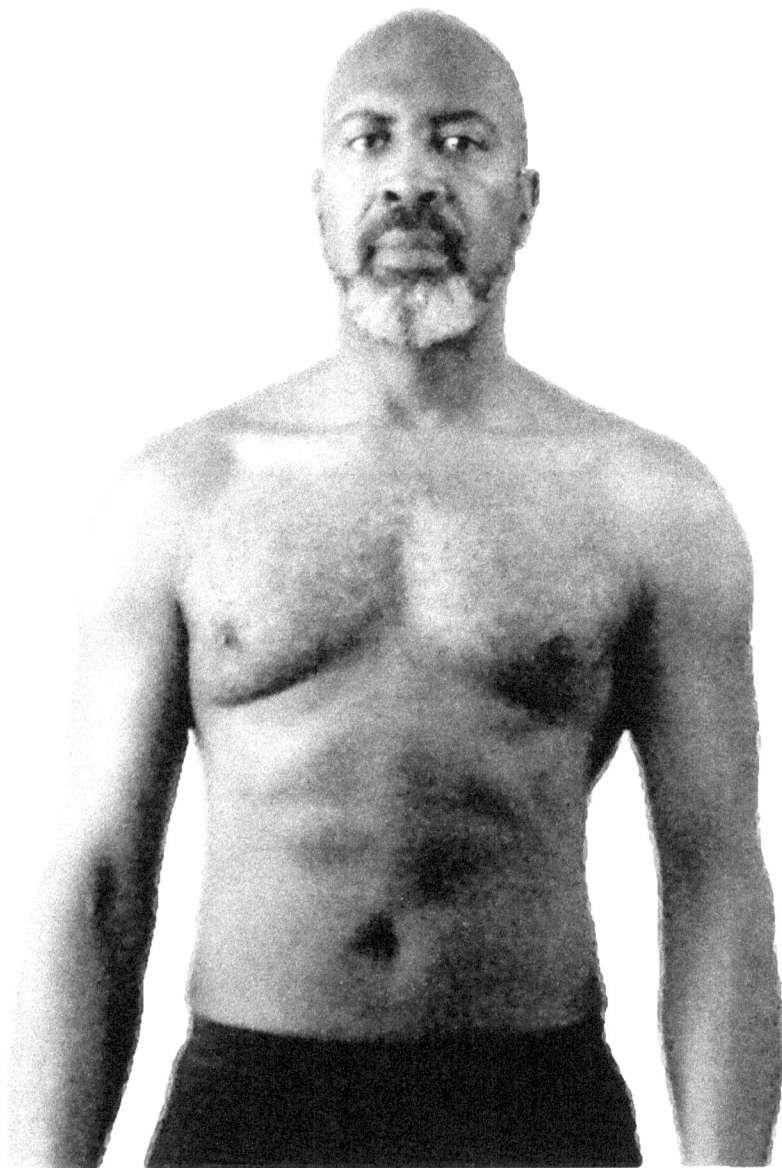

Total weight loss of 70 lbs.  36″ waist...

# 12 MONTH WEIGHT LOSS CHART

| WEEKS | M.1 | M.2 | M.3 | WK. | M.4 | M.5 | M.6 | WK. | M.7 | M.8 | M.9 | WK. | M.10 | M.11 | M.12 |
|---|---|---|---|---|---|---|---|---|---|---|---|---|---|---|---|
| Wk.1 | | | | Wk.16 | | | | Wk.31 | | | | Wk.46 | | | |
| Wk.2 | | | | Wk. 17 | | | | Wk.32 | | | | Wk.47 | | | |
| Wk.3 | | | | Wk.18 | | | | Wk.33 | | | | Wk.48 | | | |
| Wk.4 | | | | Wk.19 | | | | Wk.34 | | | | Wk.49 | | | |
| Wk.5 | | | | Wk.20 | | | | Wk.35 | | | | Wk.50 | | | |
| Wk.6 | | | | Wk.21 | | | | Wk.36 | | | | Wk.51 | | | |
| Wk.7 | | | | Wk.22 | | | | Wk.37 | | | | Wk.52 | | | |
| Wk.8 | | | | Wk.23 | | | | Wk.38 | | | | Wk.53 | | | |
| Wk.9 | | | | Wk.24 | | | | Wk.39 | | | | Wk.54 | | | |
| Wk.10 | | | | Wk.25 | | | | Wk.40 | | | | Wk.55 | | | |
| Wk.11 | | | | Wk.26 | | | | Wk.41 | | | | Wk.56 | | | |
| Wk.12 | | | | Wk.27 | | | | Wk.42 | | | | Wk.57 | | | |
| Wk.13 | | | | Wk.28 | | | | Wk.43 | | | | Wk.58 | | | |
| Wk.14 | | | | Wk.29 | | | | Wk.44 | | | | Wk.59 | | | |
| Wk.15 | | | | Wk.30 | | | | Wk.45 | | | | Wk.60 | | | |

# EXERCISE ROUTINES #1 thru #12

| DAYS | #1 | #2 | #3 | #4 | #5 | #6 | #7 | #8 | #9 | #10 | #11 | #12 | REPS | SETS |
|------|----|----|----|----|----|----|----|----|----|-----|-----|-----|------|------|
| 1 | | | | | | | | | | | | | | |
| 2 | | | | | | | | | | | | | | |
| 3 | | | | | | | | | | | | | | |
| 4 | | | | | | | | | | | | | | |
| 5 | | | | | | | | | | | | | | |
| 6 | | | | | | | | | | | | | | |
| 7 | | | | | | | | | | | | | | |
| 8 | | | | | | | | | | | | | | |
| 9 | | | | | | | | | | | | | | |
| 10 | | | | | | | | | | | | | | |
| 11 | | | | | | | | | | | | | | |
| 12 | | | | | | | | | | | | | | |
| 13 | | | | | | | | | | | | | | |
| 14 | | | | | | | | | | | | | | |
| 15 | | | | | | | | | | | | | | |

# EXERCISE ROUTINES #1 thru #12

| DAYS | #1 | #2 | #3 | #4 | #5 | #6 | #7 | #8 | #9 | #10 | #11 | #12 | REPS | SETS |
|------|----|----|----|----|----|----|----|----|----|-----|-----|-----|------|------|
| 16 | | | | | | | | | | | | | | |
| 17 | | | | | | | | | | | | | | |
| 18 | | | | | | | | | | | | | | |
| 19 | | | | | | | | | | | | | | |
| 20 | | | | | | | | | | | | | | |
| 21 | | | | | | | | | | | | | | |
| 22 | | | | | | | | | | | | | | |
| 23 | | | | | | | | | | | | | | |
| 24 | | | | | | | | | | | | | | |
| 25 | | | | | | | | | | | | | | |
| 26 | | | | | | | | | | | | | | |
| 27 | | | | | | | | | | | | | | |
| 28 | | | | | | | | | | | | | | |
| 29 | | | | | | | | | | | | | | |
| 30 | | | | | | | | | | | | | | |

www.ingramcontent.com/pod-product-compliance
Lightning Source LLC
Chambersburg PA
CBHW031500270326
41930CB00006B/173